Policies, Plans, and People

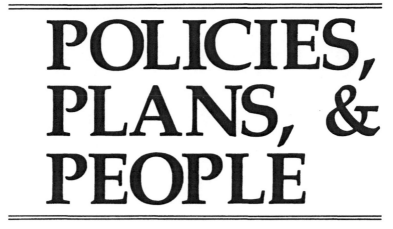

POLICIES, PLANS, & PEOPLE

Foreign Aid and Health Development

JUDITH JUSTICE

UNIVERSITY OF CALIFORNIA PRESS
Berkeley   Los Angeles   London

This book is a print-on-demand volume. It is manufactured using toner in place of ink. Type and images may be less sharp than the same material seen in traditionally printed University of California editions.

University of California Press
Berkeley and Los Angeles, California

University of California Press, Ltd.
London, England

Copyright © 1986 by The Regents of the University of California
First Paperback Printing 1989

Library of Congress Cataloging-in-Publication Data

Justice, Judith.
    Policies, plans, and people.

    (Comparative studies of health systems and medical care)
    Bibliography: p.
    Includes index.
    1. Rural health services—Nepal.   2. Health planning—Nepal.
3. Medical policy—Nepal.   4. Rural health services—Planning—International cooperation.   I. Title.   II. Series. [DNLM: 1. Anthropology, Cultural—Nepal.   2. Health Planning—Nepal.   3. Health Services—Nepal.
4. International Cooperation.   5. Primary Health Care—Nepal.   6. Public Health Administration—Nepal.   7. Rural Health—Nepal.
WA 540 JN4 J9p1]
RA771.7.N35J87   1986   362.1'09549'6   85-14161

ISBN 0-520-06788-6 (alk. paper)
Printed in the United States of America

The paper used in this publication is both acid-free and totally chlorine-free (TCF). It meets the minimum requirements of ANSI/NISO Z39.48-1992 (R 1997) (*Permanence of Paper*). ∞

Contents

Abbreviations   ix

Preface   xi

1
Introduction   1

    Nepal: The Setting   5

    Research Methods   10

2
The Health Bureaucracies: Structure and
Culture   15

    The Dynamics of Nepal's Bureaucracy   15
        Government Structure   15
        Traditional Patterns in
        Administrative Behavior   20
    The International Donor Agencies   24
        The World Health Organization
        (WHO)   25
        The United States Agency for
        International Development (USAID)   26
    Interaction Between the Government
    and the Agencies   29

Nepali Administrators and
International Advisors   35

3
Policies and Plans   46

International Health Policy and Nepal   48
Hospital-Based and Vertical Programs   48
The Shift to Integrated Basic Health
Services   51
Integrated Community Health
Program and Primary Health Care   59
The Planning Process   63
Country Health Programming   63
Further Planning Efforts   69
Planning for Community Participation:
A Case Example   74

4
Delivering Services to Rural Villages   82

A Partially Integrated Health Post   83
A Fully Integrated Health Post   88
The Local Panchayat   92
Shortages   93
The Villagers' Response to Services   95
The District Health Office   98
Problematic Roles of Health Workers   101
The Invisible Health Worker: The
Peon   101
The Community Health Volunteer and
the Village Health Worker   106

5
Sources and Channels of Information   111

Sources of Information   112
Reports   112
Field Travel   117
Formal and Informal Meetings   119

The Flow of Information within
Government   122
    Data, Plans, and Targets   122
    Vertical Barriers   125
    Horizontal Barriers   131
    Reliance on Quantitative Data   132

6
Sociocultural Information and the Health Planning
Process   135

The Anthropologist's Role in Planning
Using Sociocultural Information to
Improve Health Planning: A Case
Study   140
    Some Suggestions for Changing the
    ANM's Role   148
Overcoming Obstacles in the Health
Bureaucracy   151

Appendixes   155

    1. A Chronology of Health-Sector
       Events in Nepal   156
    2. Profile of Health Workers in ICHP   159
    3. Job Descriptions for ICHP   161
       Functions of Community Health
       Volunteer   161
       Village Health Worker   163
       Assistant Nurse-Midwife (ANM)   167

Notes   170

Bibliography   175

Index   195

Abbreviations

AID	Agency for International Development
ANM	Assistant Nurse-Midwife
BNMT	Britain Nepal Medical Trust
CDO	Chief District Officer
CEDA	Centre for Economic Development and Administration
CIDA	Canadian International Development Assistance
EPI	Expanded Program of Immunization
ESCAP	Economic and Social Commission of Asia and the Pacific
FAO	Food and Agriculture Organization
FP/MCH	Family Planning/Maternal and Child Health
HMG	His Majesty's Government of Nepal
IBHS	Integrated Basic Health Services
IBRD	International Bank for Reconstruction and Development
ICHP	Integrated Community Health Program
IDRC	International Development Research Centre
IOM	Institute of Medicine
MCH	Maternal and Child Health
MOH	Ministry of Health
NMEO	Nepal Malaria Eradication Organization
PHN	Public Health Nurse
SATA	Swiss Association for Technical Assistance

TA/DA	Travel Allowance/Daily Allowance
TBA	Traditional Birth Attendant
UNDP	United Nations Development Program
UNFPA	United Nations Fund for Population Activities
UNICEF	United Nations Children's Fund
USAID	United States Agency for International Development
VHW	Village Health Worker
WHO	World Health Organization

Preface

Although this book centers on research I carried out in Nepal during the late 1970s, it actually originated a decade earlier. My interest in the cultural aspects of foreign assistance began in the late 1960s when I was working in Africa and South Asia for international agencies. Despite the good intentions and dedication of many planners and administrators, I saw that internationally assisted health programs often resulted in services that were inappropriate to the local needs and resources, and consequently less than fully successful. Granted that foreign assistance reflects complex political and economic considerations, I thought it should be possible within these given limitations to design programs that would be culturally compatible with the populations they serve. With this end in mind, I returned to the United States to train as a medical anthropologist.

In the early 1970s in India, I also became aware that the priorities of international funding agencies shifted frequently, changing trends in international assistance. When I started my research some years later, I looked specifically at the policy then being given the highest priority—primary health care—in order to gain insight into the process through which policy trends develop and the impact they have on the national health services of countries receiving aid.

This book examines the cultural dimensions of primary

health care in Nepal, from the program's antecedents in international health policy centers in Geneva and Washington to its outcomes in remote rural villages. Drawing on extensive participant observation, I have described many features of the program that were unsuitable for the local conditions and cultures. To discover the sources of the problem, I explored the bureaucratic environments in which policymaking and planning take place, and tried to identify barriers to cultural sensitivity within the health planning process.

Although there are signs that international interest in primary health care is already waning, my recent visits to Nepal and other areas in South and Southeast Asia, as well as my further experiences as a consultant with international agencies, have confirmed that the conclusions of this study are still valid, because they refer to general processes rather than to a particular program. The intermeshing of the various actors involved in developing and implementing health programs as I observed them remains much the same today. In fact, the study's conclusions are more relevant today, because once again the priorities in international health are shifting—this time away from the integration of health services and back to a focus on specific diseases and health problems—and new cycles of policymaking and planning are under way.

My purpose in undertaking this study was to find ways for anthropologists and planners to combine their expertise in a more practical and effective approach to providing health care—in particular, to help make the tremendous monetary contributions and manpower available for assistance produce more culturally appropriate services. During the course of my research, health planners and administrators often said to me that anthropological study benefits only anthropologists, not the group being studied. I hope that my experience in international organizations and my training in the social sciences have enabled me to write a book that will be read and used by those I have studied—the foreign and Nepali health planning community—as well as by those in the academic world who are interested in the problems of development.

As yet another questioning foreigner, taking the time of

Nepali officials, I understood the burden that expatriate "helpers" place on these people. I want to thank them especially for their cooperation and for the perceptions they so freely shared with me. I am also indebted to the foreign health planners and consultants whose frankness enabled me to see the way things were in health planning. Their openness involved the risk that I would use their experience in a way that could put their work and efforts in an uncomplimentary light. I appreciate their willingness to take this risk in the interest of assisting me, and I want to reassure them and my other readers that any criticisms are directed not at individuals or groups but at organization processes. I have attempted to describe conditions and cultural forces that sometimes prevent planners from achieving their goals. I hope that the way I have organized their perceptions and my own observations and experiences will help them and their colleagues in current and future planning.

In Nepal, many people extended assistance and generous hospitality. I thank the Nepalis who shared their homes and meals and willingly provided information, even though they were often uncertain about why I was so interested in what happened at health posts and in what they did when they were ill. Their help and kindness enabled me to do this work. Over the years, officers and staff working with the international agencies in India and Nepal have provided various forms of help and hospitality. To protect their privacy and that of people mentioned in this book—villagers, health workers, government officials, and foreign planners and administrators—I have used pseudonyms for them throughout.

I want to thank the many people who have helped make this study possible by extending their encouragement, support, and friendship. My early fieldwork experience in India began under the informal tutelage of the late Wolf Ladejinsky. He shared with me his approach to understanding the realities of development by looking and listening as an observer of everyday village life. He also taught me the importance of communicating what one learns to those in decision-making positions. At the University of California at

Berkeley, Gerald Berreman helped me develop my ideas on South Asia. Leo Rose generously shared his wealth of knowledge on Nepal and the Himalayan region, in addition to his insights into South Asian government and politics. I am particularly indebted to George Foster for encouraging me to study medical anthropology and for his strong support throughout all phases of this endeavor. He gave me the benefit of his long experience by sharing his perspective on culture and health, and especially his interest in the impact of bureaucracies on health programs.

At the School of Medicine, University of California at San Francisco, Fred Dunn has made many suggestions on epidemiological points and Asian medicine, as well as directing me to excellent literature relevant to my research. Margaret Clark's pioneering work in the cultural aspects of medicine has served as a continuing inspiration. She has always been willing to talk with me about ways for anthropologists to contribute to the health field. Philip Lee of the Institute for Health Policy Studies stole time from his extremely demanding schedule to provide insight into the policy process and a stimulating exchange of ideas from the beginning of my research. He generously extended not only his own support but also support from the staff at the Institute, especially Eunice Chee, who provided calm help in frenzied moments, and Roger Black, who took on the tedious task of proofreading.

Many friends and colleagues have listened with patience and interest, and provided support in uncountable ways. My Nepali friends in Berkeley shared their personal knowledge and their well-spiced *daal bhaat*. Among other friends who have given up their valuable time to read the manuscript are Stephen Bezruchka, Dor Bahadur Bista, Ruth Dixon, Lynn Dondero, Deborah Gordon, Lynn Knauff, Anne Firth Murray, Raymond Noronha, Susan Niles, Aran Schloss, John Scholz, John Sommer, Betty Webster, and Rosemary Zumwalt. Elizabeth Nottingham prodded me into writing at the difficult stage of starting a book. I am grateful to Joan Bentley, who always made time in her busy life to give detailed comments on the manuscript drawing on her extensive knowledge and experience of nursing and health training in

Nepal. Duane Smith helped me understand the perspective of health planners with his probing questions, his honest response to my writing, his openness to discussing the difficulties of the planner's role, and his willingness to explore the contributions anthropologists can make. Shri Kul Shekhar Sharma and Dr. Ram Prakash Yadav made invaluable suggestions on the final draft.

I thank the faculty and students at the Centre for Nepal and Asian Studies, Tribhuvan University, where I was a visiting Research Scholar, for their assistance. I am grateful for research funds provided by the National Institute of General Medical Sciences, National Institutes of Health.

Without Charles Leslie's early interest in my research and his insistence that I publish it, not to mention his sharp editorial eye, this study would not have developed into a book. Ellen Hershey's assistance has gone beyond that of an editor. In hours of discussing my experiences and ideas, she helped me bring forward and express my thoughts in book form. She worked with me to achieve a more vigorous style, knowing that I wanted to reach out beyond the academic culture to planners and administrators who are working in the field.

I thank my parents for their support and caring over the years. They have patiently accepted the extra burden of worry placed on them by a daughter who travels to unfamiliar parts of the world so far away.

This book is dedicated to Elizabeth Colson, who has been my teacher, mentor, and friend, guiding me through every phase of the research and writing. She treated me to a lively exchange of ideas while walking with me up and down the Berkeley hills, getting me in physical and intellectual shape for the Himalayas. She has inspired and encouraged me with her steadfast belief in the importance of addressing policy issues forthrightly.

Berkeley, California   Judith Justice
July 1985

1

Introduction

The relationship between planning and performance can be perplexing, even in simple situations where few people are involved. It becomes much more complicated when plans are made on a vast scale for the benefit of people whom the planners themselves may never meet and whose view of their own most pressing needs may never be asked. How can the gap between the people on the receiving end of planning and the well-intentioned designs of planners often far removed from the recipients best be bridged, so that imagination and resources may achieve the most beneficial result?

Since the 1940s international health agencies, in cooperation with national governments, have achieved some remarkable successes in developing hospital-based health services and in attacking communicable diseases. The worldwide eradication of smallpox presents the most dramatic example of what has been accomplished through international expertise and technical assistance. The incidence of malaria has been checked, though not eradicated, and health conditions in general have improved considerably. During the 1960s, however, international attention focused on the rapidly growing need to extend basic health services, both preventive and curative, to more people, and especially to rural populations in developing countries. The new approaches designed to meet this need—originally called basic health services and now called primary health care—require close, long-term relationships between health care providers and rural communities. Unlike smallpox and malaria workers, who could arrive in a village, conduct an immunization clinic or spray with DDT, and then leave, the primary health care worker must live in the village, establish bonds of trust, and work with the villagers to introduce more healthful behavioral patterns. In short, he must become part of the community.

Thus, international health efforts have entered a new era, one in which the efficient application of technical expertise alone is not sufficient. The shift has been difficult to make. All too often the massive infusion of effort and funding from international health agencies has had disappointing results at the grass roots level. Health planners and administrators generally acknowledge that their policies and plans have not always produced effective services, in part because social and cultural information about the people to be served has not received adequate attention. Although awareness of the links between health and social dimensions has been increasing, taking social and cultural variables into account is by no means an easy matter. In recent years international agencies have been attempting to accomplish this by working closely with the national governments concerned and by hiring social scientists to advise them on the social and cultural appropriateness of their plans. But these attempts have yet to produce a noticeable improvement in the health services provided in many rural areas.

My own interest in the use of social and cultural information in health planning has been developing for more than fifteen years. It started during my first experiences as a program officer with training in public health and community development for United Nations agencies; it intensified during my research as an anthropologist; and it has broadened during my recent work as a consultant on primary health care for international health agencies.

This book began with the frustrations I experienced in 1973–75 when administering a large nutrition education program in India. Planned by the Food and Agriculture Organization (FAO) in Rome and the United Nations Children's Fund (UNICEF) in New York, the program was implemented by the Indian government. I quickly realized that although it was well intentioned, it was ill suited to the social and cultural realities of Indian life at that time. Yet there has been a great deal of social science research in India. The cultural patterns of virtually every major group in the population have been studied by both Indian and foreign researchers. Furthermore, a vast literature—much of it based on the Indian experience—exists on health-related behavior and on the problems resulting from the introduction of modern medical technology in developing countries.

I wondered why this information had not been used to plan a program that would be more appropriate to Indian culture. Perhaps the information had not been made available to planners at the right time or in the right way. No doubt different kinds of information would be needed at the various levels and stages of planning. If social scientists knew more about what planners needed and how to present their findings, could their information be more effective? Of course, many factors—notably, economic and political considerations—shape health policies and plans, but within these parameters there should be ways for planners to take social and cultural realities into account.

In order to discover what kinds of information planners needed and at what stage in planning they needed it, I decided to investigate Nepal's rural health program, officially known as the Integrated Community Health Program (ICHP). I selected Nepal as a testing ground because it was in the Asian area with which I was already familiar and also because it was a recent and important focus for international agencies in primary health care. Since primary health care was being presented by international policymakers as the most socially sensitive approach to serving rural areas, it seemed to me that planners would need social and cultural information about rural Nepal.

Nepal had already adopted an Integrated Community Health Program that was initially designed to combine five existing "vertical" (disease-specific) health programs—smallpox, malaria, leprosy, tuberculosis, and family planning/maternal and child health—to forge a community health structure for providing basic health services. During the late 1970s, ICHP was gradually being transformed into primary health care, which provided an opportunity to study planning and implementation during the transitional phase. I examined ICHP in 1977–79 from the top down—that is, from its international antecedents to the village level—to find out to what extent social and cultural information was used in its planning. By studying its implementation, I was able to compare the plan formulated by Nepali and foreign planners with the results at the grass roots level and to evaluate its cultural appropriateness.

My earlier observations in India were repeated in the first stages of this new research. Most health planners dealing with Nepal were not seeking social and cultural information, nor did they consider it necessary. More significant, they did not appear to be influenced by what they already did know about social and cultural conditions. Why weren't they?

This question prompted me to extend my research beyond the kinds of information health planners needed to the planning environment itself, in order to see whether there were barriers to using information about local conditions in planning at the national and international levels. How do the bureaucratic cultures in which planning takes place affect the way planners perceive and use information about the people they are trying to serve?

In attempting to study the culture of a health planning bureaucracy, one enters terrain largely unexplored by anthropologists. Although the recent anthropological literature reflects a growing recognition of bureaucracies as social and cultural systems and provides a number of studies of complex organizations,[1] anthropologists working on bureaucracies have yet to develop a strong theoretical tradition. Few guidelines exist for studies in this emergent field. A growing body of literature by political scientists on the politics of non-Western societies focuses on bureaucracies as administrative structures and on the bureaucrats themselves (Rose and Landau 1977). Much of the sociological literature on bureaucracies is addressed not to the culture of bureaucracies but rather to their structure. I am dealing with both the Nepali and international bureaucracies as cultural systems. This study thus contributes to a new anthropology dealing with one of the major institutions now influencing our lives—the multinational organization, with its own goals and culture.

Nepal: The Setting

Nepal lies in the central Himalayas, wedged between India and China (see map 1). A small country, some 500 miles long and no more than 110 miles wide, it has a population of approximately 14 million.* The flat Terai plains in the south, the central hills, and the high Himalayas in the north divide the country into three areas. The Kosi, Karnali, and Gandaki river systems, which traverse it from north to south, are uncrossable when swollen by monsoon rains and melting snows, as they are during much of the year. The mountainous terrain and distinct geographic divisions isolate the rural areas from the central government in Kathmandu Valley and have hindered the development of transportation, communication, and other infrastructures, including health facilities. Ninety-six percent of the population lives in rural areas, most of which are so inaccessible from Kathmandu that they can be reached only by walking for hours or even days along steep, winding trails.

Nepal has few natural resources. Although 90 percent of the population depends on agriculture for a living, only 12 percent of the land is arable. Declining soil fertility, erosion, and variable climatic conditions complicate agricultural development. Food, fodder, and firewood are scarce in the hills and mountains, where 60 percent of the population lives. Because of increasing deforestation, firewood is becoming even more scarce, and overgrazing has exacerbated erosion. Drinking water is polluted in many areas and often must be carried long distances.

The annual per capita income is $120, among the lowest in the world, and in the hill communities it is estimated to

---

*Statistical data cited in this book describe conditions at the time of the research in 1978-79.

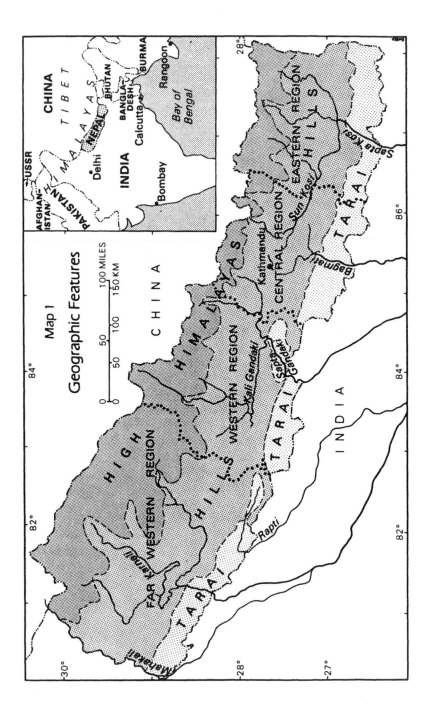

Map 1

Geographic Features

be only $25 (World Bank 1978:2). Since most of the population lives at a subsistence level, landholdings are a more significant indication of the standard of living than income. The average family in the Nepali hills has only one acre of arable land, even less than the average family in Bangladesh (Rose and Scholz 1980:94). The population comprises approximately 75 ethnic groups, and more than thirty languages are spoken. Eighty-one percent of the population is illiterate. Although officially a Hindu kingdom, Nepal has religious diversity, with substantial Buddhist and Muslim minorities in certain areas. Thus, rural isolation, poverty, and illiteracy along with linguistic, ethnic, and religious divisions hinder the extension of government services.

While much has been accomplished in Nepal in combating some diseases (for example, smallpox and malaria), morbidity and mortality rates are still very high, especially for infants and children. Childhood diseases constitute the country's major health problem. Although the accuracy of available statistics is questionable, it is estimated that 54 percent of all deaths are among children under five and that between 134 and 260 infants per 1,000 live births die in their first year, one of the highest rates in Asia. Because of the high infant mortality rate, life expectancy at birth is low: 46 years for males, 43 for females (Nepal Ministry of Health 1979).

The main causes of infant and child death are diarrhea from impure water and foodborne diseases, nutritional deficiencies, chest infections, other communicable diseases, and accidents. Many of these diseases are preventable, as are the major causes of adult death, which include communicable diseases such as malaria, leprosy, and tuberculosis; accidents; and maternity-related diseases. Maternal morbidity and mortality, which rank second among Nepal's major health problems, are caused by poor nutrition, frequent pregnancies, lack of proper prenatal care, complications of pregnancy and delivery, and medically unsupervised abortions (UNICEF 1978). Nepal's crude birthrate per 1,000 population, estimated from the 1976 National Fertility Survey, was 43.6—again, one of the highest in Asia.

Until the early 1950s most health care was provided by family members and indigenous practitioners of several kinds, including herbalists and spiritualists. A multiplicity of medical traditions still exists in Nepal, and these traditions are used interchangeably and in varying combinations. *Jharfuknes, jhankris,* and *dhamis* exorcise evil spirits with a combination of chants, mantras, drumbeating, and animal sacrifices. Buddhist lamas use prayers to avert catastrophe. Ayurvedic specialists practice Hindu herbal medicine. Practitioners of homeopathy, acupuncture, Yunani (Greco-Arabic medicine), and Tibetan medicine are also available. Traditional midwives—*sudenis* and *dhais*—attend births in some regions. Among the traditional practitioners, however, only the government-trained Ayurvedic doctors *(Vaidya* and *Kabiraj)* are officially recognized and supported by the government.[2]

Western scientific medicine—or allopathic medicine, as it is called throughout South Asia—came to Nepal relatively late. Unlike other South Asian countries (Sri Lanka, Pakistan, Bangladesh, and India), Nepal was never colonized. It remained closed to most outsiders and to foreign health systems until 1951, when a revolution restored the monarchy and led to the opening of the international airport at Kathmandu.

International health assistance soon followed, provided first by a number of Christian missions, foundations, and trusts. By 1951, Nepal had a few mission and government hospitals, located mainly in Kathmandu Valley. It also had twelve Nepali physicians trained abroad in allopathic medicine, along with some paramedical assistants who dispensed medications, gave injections, and dressed wounds (USAID 1975:8). During this period, Indian and other foreign drug firms began to promote allopathic drugs. In 1954, India, the United States, and the World Health Organization (WHO) were among the first external donors to give assistance to Nepal for health-related activities. The Soviet Union and China were also early contributors.

With technical advice and financial assistance from various external sources, a government health system was organized and expanded by the newly formed Ministry of Health. In 1956, planned development of health services began with the government's first five-year development plan. Between the 1950s and the late 1970s, Nepal expanded its health services to include nearly 70 hospitals with 15 to 300 beds each; approximately 450 medical doctors, of whom only 25 percent are located in rural areas; 350 nurses, with 14 percent in rural areas; and 550 health posts, staffed by paramedical workers and distributed throughout Nepal's 75 districts.

By 1978, despite the impressive gains made by several disease-specific programs and in the expansion of hospital-based services, broad community health needs in Nepal were still only partially being met, especially in mountainous rural areas remote from Kathmandu. The health budget was largely consumed in providing hospital services that served urban people, who made up only 4 percent of the total population. Over 50 percent of the country's 1,500 hospital beds were located in Kathmandu, and most rural hospitals were small fifteen-bed units that were relatively expensive to equip and staff, and unable to provide comprehensive hospital services (World Bank 1978:18). Rural health facilities were generally understaffed, undersupplied, and underutilized. Because the health service system did not tackle the underlying causes of illness, such as poor nutrition, polluted water, and lack of education in hygiene and sanitation, scarce resources were being inefficiently used (World Bank 1978:18).

In addition to the obvious need for health services, Nepal's strategic location between two major Third World powers, its political neutrality and stability, its poverty, and its beauty make it an attractive focus for international health aid. During the past twenty-five years, the number of donors has multiplied. In April 1979, thirty-seven donors[3] were contributing funds and/or equipment and personnel for health purposes (Health Associates 1979).

With so many donors operating in Nepal, aid-assisted programs inevitably overlap. In some instances, donors have cooperated in funding and staffing particular projects. Malaria eradication, for example, is funded by both the World Health Organization (WHO) and the United States Agency for International Development (USAID). The rural health program, the focus of this study, was being funded jointly by at least fifteen agencies in 1978–79. It had two major donors, however: WHO and USAID. They regarded it as a test case of how to bring about the integration of the vertical projects to provide basic health services, and subsequently, to incorporate the concept of primary health care—a high priority among international health policymakers.

Research Methods

To examine the planning and implementation of primary health care in Nepal, I started at the international level and progressed to the delivery of services at the local level, the rural Nepali village. By using traditional anthropological methods—in-depth, open-ended interviewing and participant observation—I studied the activities of international planners involved with Nepal, the formulation of government priorities and programs in Kathmandu, and the delivery of health services in outlying districts and villages. Because Nepal is a small country with relatively centralized decision making at the national level, it was possible to trace the flow of information between the international, national, and local levels.

The first research challenge was to gain access to the bureaucracies in order to understand how planners work and how their perceptions and social interactions influence the decisions they make. My previous experience of working in international agencies (one year with the United Nations in New York and two years with UNICEF in India) had provided me with some understanding of the internal structure of international aid agencies and of how these agencies interact with national governments.

In July 1976, I visited the headquarters of several international aid agencies and foundations in New York and Washington to interview staff about official priorities with respect to health, the utilization of local health resources in the projects they sponsored, and the assistance they gave to South Asian countries. These exploratory visits gave me some understanding of the genesis of international health policy as well as confidence that it would be possible to obtain the agencies' cooperation.

I spent seven weeks in Nepal in July and August 1977, primarily to study the Nepali language and to carry out some preliminary research on the Nepal government's priorities and programs in health. I also met with field staff members of various international organizations to discuss their support for Nepal's health programs and to learn how they adapted international policy to the Nepal government's priorities. This short visit was very useful, for it enabled me to meet many of the officials concerned with health services in Nepal and to become acquainted with some of the background documentation for the rural health program.

In order to find out who the planners were and how they worked, I made contact with the major international agencies supporting rural health programs in Nepal in 1978, including WHO in Geneva and New Delhi, UNICEF and the United Nations Development Program (UNDP) in New York, USAID and the World Bank in Washington, the Canadian International Development Agency (CIDA) and the International Research Development Centre (IDRC) in Ottawa, the Britain Nepal Medical Trust (BNMT), the Dooley Foundation, and consulting groups contracted for the Integrated Community Health Program under USAID.

I visited the headquarters of these agencies in May and June 1978 on my way to Nepal to review documentation and interview staff members who formulated agency health policy or were associated with work in Nepal. I also interviewed staff social scientists. I wanted to find out from them what their roles had been in planning the donor agency's assistance to Nepal's health program and what kinds of social and cultural data had been available.

From June through September 1978, I interviewed Nepali officials in the Ministry of Finance, the Planning Commission, and the Ministry and Department of Health in Kathmandu, including people employed in ICHP and other health programs. I met with people who had worked on Nepal's long-term health plans as well as those implementing integrated health services. I also interviewed staff members and consultants with the various international agencies and reviewed available documents.

In order to understand the actual workings of ICHP in Nepal, I interviewed government officials, administrative health officers, health service practitioners, and patients, and observed activities at the district and health post levels over a period of twelve months. For this last step, I made trips to ten districts that had different geographical characteristics and represented different phases of ICHP: Surkhet in the far west; Palpa and Kaski in the west; Dhading in the central region; Lalitpur in Kathmandu Valley; Sankhuwasabha and Dhankuta in the east; and Parsa, Bara, and Rautahat in the Terai, the southern plains (see Map 2). During these visits I familiarized myself with government activities at the district level, with the role of the local and district *panchayats* (government councils) and health post committees, with health facilities, and with the local operation of ICHP.

In addition to interviewing health officers and administrative officials in the district centers, I visited twenty-four health posts to meet health workers and patients using the services. It took me several days of walking to reach many of these locations. I spent a number of days at each post, accompanied village health workers on their home visits, and made follow-up visits to the homes of patients who came to the posts. I also visited several small community projects sponsored on a pilot basis by religious missions and voluntary organizations. On some of these field visits I was alone or with my Nepali research assistant, a Thakali from the western hills. On others I was accompanied by local health workers, by officials from the central or district level, or by foreign health advisors. The latter visits enabled me to understand what kind of information health officials sought and how they obtained it. By moving back and forth from the local to the national level, I was able to observe how information was transmitted in both directions and what factors facilitated or constrained the flow. Although I tried to understand the functioning of the health programs

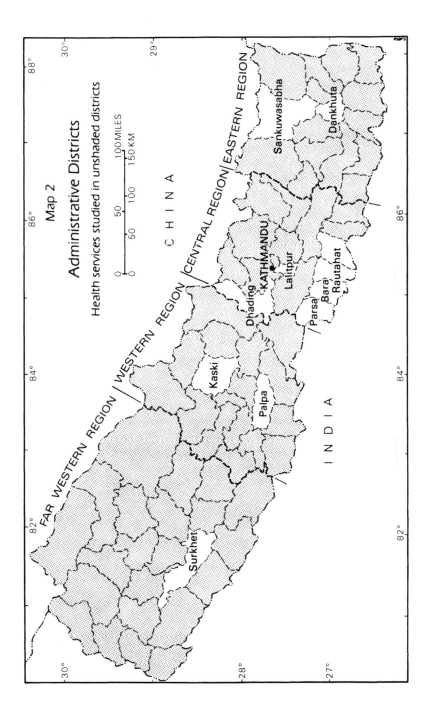

Map 2

Administrative Districts

Health services studied in unshaded districts

CHINA

INDIA

FAR WESTERN REGION | WESTERN REGION | CENTRAL REGION | EASTERN REGION

Surkhet

Kaski

Palpa

Dhading

KATHMANDU

Lalitpur

Parsa

Bara

Rautahat

Sankuwasabha

Dankhuta

0   50   100
0   50   100   150 KM
100 MILES

I observed, I was not in a position to evaluate their medical effectiveness, and this was not my intention. My aim was to see how appropriate these programs were to the local culture.

By visiting rural health posts and accompanying health workers on their daily rounds, I acquired some understanding of local conditions and of the problems faced by health workers, usually of urban origin, in an isolated rural environment. The difficulties of travel and communication made me more sensitive to the obstacles faced by Nepali and foreign planners based in Kathmandu in obtaining information from the local level.

During my research, my original question—What kinds of information do planners need, and when do they need it?—evolved into the question, What contribution can an anthropologist make to health planning? The answer must come from an understanding of the planning process—the complex cultural settings in which policies and plans are made and applied, how these settings affect the planner's priorities and point of view, and how policies and plans filter down through stages of implementation to interact with cultures at the local level. Using the traditional anthropological approach of studying a culture through the perceptions of participants, I hoped to enhance our understanding of this process and thus to find more effective ways of assisting planners in their difficult undertaking of designing programs that will eventually provide services for all.

2

The Health Bureaucracies: Structure and Culture

Understanding the Integrated Health Program requires a look at the organizations that created it: the Nepal government and the international donor agencies. Their goals, structure, and patterns of operation have determined how ICHP was planned and carried out. Cultural differences among the health bureaucracies complicate the planning process: thus, the program that has emerged reflects the interactions among the bureaucratic cultures as well as their linkages to the cultures of rural Nepal.

The Dynamics of Nepal's Bureaucracy

Government Structure

Since 1951, Nepal has been governed by a constitutional monarchy. Broadly speaking, Nepal's administrative bureaucracy consists of three levels, with the king and the Palace Secretariat at the top. The king is the chief figure in policy formulation. In the 1970s, all formal channels of communication converged in the Palace Secretariat, which consisted of the king's secretaries and assistants. This was the major policymaking institution in the government, but it had a less important role in implementing policy.* An important part of the Palace Secretariat at that time was the Janch Bhuj Kendra (the Centre for Enquiry and Investigation), which consisted mainly of handpicked bureaucrats who formulated programs under direct Palace Secretariat supervision. This body worked on special assignments, assisted by experts from relevant ministries. For example, two doctors from the Ministry of Health and an official from the Ministry of Finance were temporarily seconded for nine months to the Janch Bhuj Kendra to prepare the Long-Term Health Plan, which was released in 1975.

At the second administrative level is the Central Secretariat, which consists of the ministries and departments. Although less directly involved in defining policy, the Central Secretariat gathers and provides data for the Palace Secretariat and the king, and it is directly responsible for implementing policy decisions.

The district and local administrations form the third level. Nepal is divided into fourteen zones, each of them headed by a zonal commissioner for administrative purposes. The zonal commissioner is appointed by the king and reports directly to the Palace but has marginal administrative powers. The zones are further divided into districts, seventy-five in all, with each headed by a chief district officer (CDO) who works under the Home Ministry. The CDO is responsible for maintaining law and order and for coordinating all development and social welfare activities, including those pertaining to health. District officers are formally part of the national public service and are responsible to the Central Secretariat.

In 1978 the expression of local interests was provided for by a four-level system of elected government councils called *panchayats*. In 1962, after a brief experiment with a system

---

*This account describes the government structure at the time of my research during 1978–79. Major changes in Nepal's political process, including direct election to the National Panchayat, have occurred since 1979, but their effects on health planning, if any, cannot yet be determined.

of parliamentary democracy, King Mahendra introduced a partyless political system based on village panchayats, district panchayats, zonal assemblies, and the national panchayat, Nepal's legislative body. The Council of Ministers, or cabinet, the executive organization, was appointed by the king from the national panchayat (Bhooshan 1979:39).

Health policies are implemented by the Ministry of Health (one of the ministries within the Central Secretariat), headed by the Minister of Health (Fig. 1). Directly under the Minister is the Secretary of Health, who is the chief administrator of all Ministry of Health activities, and under the Secretary is the Department of Health Services, headed by the Director-General of Health Services. The Integrated Community Health Program was one of several programs administered by the Department of Health Services in 1978. While the other programs were single-purpose mass campaigns, ICHP was designed to deliver all types of health care services— curative, preventive, and promotive. According to long-term plans, by 1985 all single-purpose or vertical programs, such as the malaria and tuberculosis programs, were to be integrated into ICHP. ICHP was perceived as the support structure for primary health care, through its aid to and collaboration with the community at all levels of its operation.

The central division of ICHP in Kathmandu was headed by a senior public health administrator, a medical doctor, who was directly responsible to the Director-General of Health Services. This administrator, more commonly referred to as the project chief, dealt with all matters in the ICHP program and coordinated efforts with other government departments and international donor agencies. Two senior medical officers assisted the chief of ICHP and were in charge of its routine management.

At the local level, ICHP was administered by district health offices, each headed by a district medical officer, and services were provided by staff at the village health posts. In practice, the health inspector, who reported to the medical officer, supervised district public health activities, including health post operations.

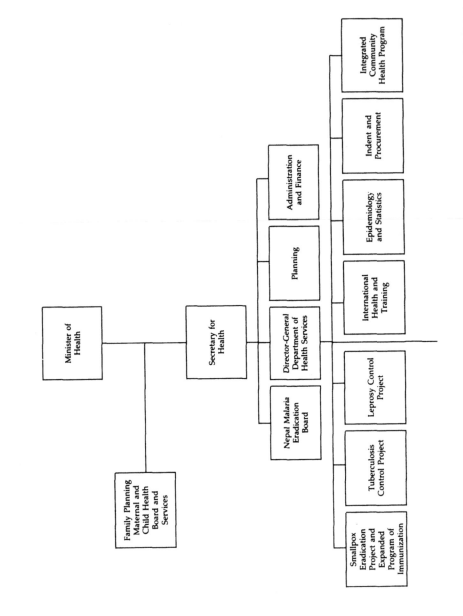

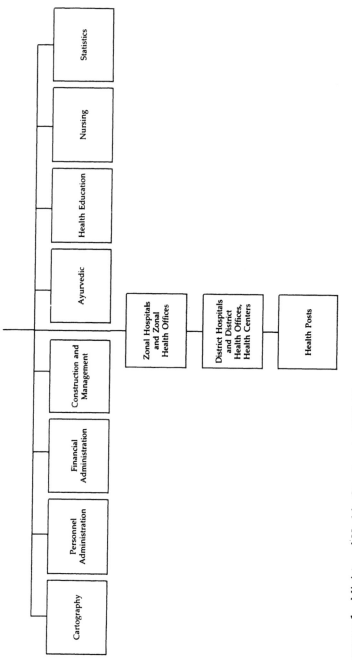

FIGURE 1 *Ministry of Health: Structure in 1978–79.*

Traditional Patterns in Administrative Behavior

The Nepali system of government presents an orderly progression of channels for information and power from the elected panchayats at the village, district, zonal, and national levels to the king and policymaking bodies at the top, and back down through the ministries to the administrative structure that carries out policy at the district and village levels. Certainly it is a system whose architecture, at least in rough outline, seems straightforward enough to foreigners working in Nepal. However, it cannot be understood apart from the broader context of Nepal's political history and culture, for although the country is small, regional differences influence relations with the centralized government. And alongside the formal bureaucratic structure, there exist complex, deeply rooted informal networks based on regional identities, ethnic and caste distinctions, and family ties that still exert powerful influences on how things are done.

Regionalism has its roots in the country's origins. At one time the area that is now Nepal consisted of about fifty small, separately ruled principalities inhabited by various caste and ethnic groups. In the last half of the eighteenth century, Prithvi Narayan Shah combined these states into a unified political and social system, although some of the former rulers continued to govern their territories for a time under the Shah dynasty's direction (Bhooshan 1979:40). In 1770 the Shah dynasty moved its capital from Gorkha, in the western hills, to the central Kathmandu Valley, formerly referred to as Nepal, and expanded its central authority throughout the realm. Thus, Nepal became a unified nation-state more than 200 years ago. Yet the legacy of the original Himalayan states remains, for Nepal is still a country of discrete communities and villages, with marked differences between the central culture in Kathmandu and the many local cultures at the district and village levels. Even within regions, there are several ethnic groups with different languages, customs, and political cultures (Scholz 1981:2).

Based on ethnic differences and the caste system, the traditional Nepali cultures were rigidly hierarchical. From 1770 to 1846, elite families and their allies dominated politics at the central level: "It was during this period that familial alliance systems (chakari), under which several client elite families were affiliated with a faction led by a noble family, emerged as a normal feature of Nepali politics" (Rose and Scholz 1980:23).

From 1846 to 1951, Nepal's isolation from external economic and political influences was exaggerated under the authoritarian rule of the Rana family, and Nepal during this period has sometimes been described as a feudal state. The century of isolation was abruptly ended by the 1951 revolution, which restored the Shah dynasty kings to power. Since then, tremendous change has taken place as political and administrative institutions have been recognized to meet the demands of a developing nation. Foreign assistance agencies have attempted to export to Nepal the principles of "administration, management, and organization based upon Western concepts of efficiency, economy and rational decision-making" (Rose and Landau 1977:42–43) through administrative advisors from India, the United States, and the United Nations (Goodall 1963, 1966), and through the education of Nepali bureaucrats in Western-style institutions in public administration and related fields.[1]

Despite this program of modernization, traditional patterns of social interaction, characterized by kinship ties, patron-client relations, caste hierarchy, and regional and ethnic identities, have endured and continue to underlie Nepali politics and administration today. The Nepali system remains hierarchical, with certain elite families having special privileges and responsibilities. Thus, in the central government, most of the high offices are held by members of elite Brahman, Chetri, and Newar families. Allegiance to one's family remains a strong social value, and favoritism toward family members is an expected form of behavior.

The legacy of the chakari system remains in extended family alliances, under which most of the leading families still have a number of client families with a long history of interaction and interdependence. High officials in the bureaucracy are still expected to protect and promote their clients, who return political loyalty to their patrons. Much of the rotation of jobs within the bureaucracy can be understood only within the context of family and other social relations (Rose and Landau 1977:48).

In addition to the official channels provided by government, then, information and power in the Nepali system often move along networks created by social and cultural traditions. Traditional networks also play a key role in linking Nepal's diverse local cultures with the center. As discussed, some 96 percent of Nepal's population lives in small villages. The transmittal of information about villagers' needs to the central bureaucracy, and conversely, the local implementation of central policies and programs, depend on the linkages between the central and local levels. Historically, local elite families have bridged the gap. Local elites, who play only a minor role in central politics, are a critical force at the district and local levels because of their capacity to promote or resist the implementation of central government policies along lines that serve their interests (Rose and Scholz 1980:24). Thus, Nepal's bureaucracy, although influenced by Western organizational concepts, must respond to local demands that are still strongly determined by traditional political cultures.

The elites' role as intermediaries came about during the Rana period, from 1846 to 1951, when central and district government procedures were standardized. To link villages and the central bureaucracy, local elites were recruited into the government revenue hierarchy. Because village cultures remained isolated, and because the Ranas minimized contact and competition among local elites, the linkages between villages and the central bureaucracy depended mostly on a clearly defined status hierarchy of face-to-face relationships (Scholz 1981:13).

Changes were introduced in the local political culture after 1951 through the dominant role of the monarchy, the introduction of political parties, and the establishment of the panchayat system and developmental bureaucracy. Local elites, especially Brahman and Chetri lineages and Kathmandu-based Newar families, with traditional family alliances, retained positions in the new networks, but they were less secure because their relationship with the central institutions had become increasingly complex.

The development of political parties in the 1950s offered local elites their first opportunity to participate directly in central political institutions, and in the process established links between villages and Kathmandu that were more direct and responsive to local problems than were the official administrative channels (Rose and Scholz 1980:83–91). In the 1960s the introduction of the partyless panchayat system created the opportunity for new networks among local elites, although in many areas the old alliances still predominate (Scholz 1981:21).

Contact with the central bureaucracy is a continuing problem for local-level groups and still depends on networks based on family, lineage, party, and panchayat relationships. The advent of a specialized civil service to administer the rapidly growing development programs, financed mainly by foreign aid, has expanded government services into districts and further affected relations between the local and central levels. Although new communication channels have been established between local elites and district officials, many elites still find direct, informal interaction with personal and family contacts in Kathmandu more effective for solving village problems than dealing with intermediaries through the official channels.[2]

These same informal networks link rural villages with the central health bureaucracy. Before 1951 there was no central health bureaucracy, since health care depended on a few hospitals in urban areas and traditional medical practitioners in local communities. After 1951 the government started to introduce national health programs that extended to the local level, beginning with malaria and smallpox programs, and then establishing district health centers and village health posts. By the late 1970s, community participation was being encouraged through district and village health committees composed of local representatives and panchayats. Thus, local elites became the intermediaries for health programs between culturally remote villagers and the central bureaucracy, transmitting information about local needs and obtaining services. In this process, however, where and how services were provided often reflected the priorities of the elite intermediaries more than those of the general population.

The International Donor Agencies

The donor agencies operating in the international health field include multilateral agencies, bilateral agencies, and private foundations and voluntary organizations. Multilateral agencies are staffed by nationals of many countries, reflecting the international sources of their funds. Among these, the most prominent is the World Health Organization (WHO), the major United Nations agency in health. Bilateral or binational agencies involve only two countries, those of the donor and the recipient. The United States Agency for International Development (USAID) is among the largest bilateral contributors. Voluntary organizations and foundations have private funding, and they may draw their funds and staff from one or many countries. Secular private agencies giving international grants to many countries for health services include the Ford and Rockefeller foundations as well as smaller organizations, such as Oxfam and Save the Children. Catholic and Protestant mission organizations also provide health services in many developing countries.

At least fifteen multilateral, bilateral, and voluntary agencies contributed to the Integrated Community Health Program, which depended largely on foreign sources for financial support as well as for technical advice.[3] The largest and most influential of these were WHO and USAID. How do these organizations operate, and how was their presence felt in Nepal in the late 1970s?

The World Health Organization (WHO)

The World Health Organization was established in 1946, its objective being "the attainment by all people of the highest possible level of health" (Basch 1978:358). Policy is determined by the Annual World Health Assembly, which is attended by delegates of all member countries. WHO's work falls into two major categories: services to governments, which take the form of projects carried out in member countries at their request; and central technical services, which include providing epidemiological services, coordinating policy on health aspects of travel and commerce, establishing standards for vaccines and pharmaceuticals, and disseminating information through meetings and educational and publishing efforts (Basch 1978:359). Mass campaigns against specific diseases were the chief focus of WHO's early years. This strategy met with spectacular success in eradicating smallpox in the 1970s and significantly reduced the incidence of malaria, among other achievements. During the 1970s, WHO turned its efforts toward increasing access to comprehensive health services, especially for rural populations in developing countries.

The headquarters for WHO is located in Geneva. Its six regional offices and many country offices work closely with national ministries of health to provide technical assistance to country health activities and to coordinate WHO-supported field projects. To support its worldwide activities, WHO had grown by 1975 to a major international organization, with a staff of more than 5,500 people and a regular budget of U.S. $147 million, with additional funds for research and special programs. Some field projects are funded jointly by WHO and other sources, such as the country concerned, other United Nations agencies, and bilateral agencies (Basch 1978:358).

The WHO country office in Nepal, located in Kathmandu, reports to the regional office for Southeast Asia located in New Delhi. The Nepal country office consists of a country representative, a deputy representative, Nepali support staff, and long- and short-term consultants and advisors assigned to specific projects, such as ICHP. The country office works directly with Nepal's Ministry of Health, mainly by providing educational fellowships, sponsoring meetings and workshops, and giving professional and technical assistance through consultants and advisors.

Because of its early focus on combating specific diseases, WHO emphasizes medical expertise. In Nepal's country office, as in others, many professional WHO staff members are physicians. The country representative in 1978–79 was a European physician, supported by a deputy representative, a physician from Asia. WHO's thirteen foreign consultants (from several different countries) worked in a wide range of areas, including malaria eradication, leprosy control, water and sanitation, laboratory services, training programs for health personnel, and health planning. The country office was frequently visited by staff and consultants from both the regional office and from the Geneva headquarters. In addition to providing technical advice, some consultants and staff members came specifically for country or regional meetings sponsored and financed by WHO.

WHO was the second most active donor agency for ICHP. Staff members working directly with the program included three physicians: one advised on the integrated approach; another on immunization activities; and the third on high-level health planning. Although these advisors all shared a medical background, they had widely different cultural backgrounds (Asian, West European, and Russian).

The United States Agency for International Development (USAID)

USAID is the largest bilateral donor of health aid to developing countries, including Nepal. Its policy guidelines originate in the U.S. Congress, the U.S. Department of State, and the Policy Division of USAID. The agency is therefore accountable to all three levels. Although USAID's structure and personnel practices are established in Washington, the bureaucracy is decentralized, with country missions in recipient countries. Washington relies on these distant missions for information, which is transmitted through the country "desk," located in the appropriate regional subdivision of the Washington office.

In Nepal, USAID has been actively involved in health planning and vertical programs, especially the family planning and malaria programs, as well as being the primary donor to ICHP. Between 1976 and 1979 it contributed almost $3 million to ICHP: some $2 million for technical assistance, commodities, and training, and about $1 million for local currency budget support, workshops, and locally procured commodities (American Public Health Association 1980:34). In general, USAID's assistance takes a different form than WHO's, which is restricted primarily to providing technical assistance at the ministerial level. While USAID works with the Ministry of Health, it also provides more financial and technical assistance to functioning field programs. Very generally speaking, Nepalis describe WHO as providing advice at the policy and planning levels and USAID as providing resources for implementation—funds, equipment and supplies, and advice.

In 1978–79, USAID maintained a large administrative and support staff in Nepal, consisting of twenty-five Americans and fifty Nepalis, who handled all assistance for agriculture, education, and so on, as well as for health. Only two Americans and two Nepalis on the regular staff worked directly on health programs, however. The USAID Health and Family Planning Section was headed by AID's Health Officer, a physician with previous experience in Asia, who was assisted by a former Peace Corps volunteer with public health training.

In addition to its regular staff, USAID has had both long- and short-term advisors in Nepal. Several short-term consultants came from the United States in 1978–79: among others, a group to prepare economic, social, and budgetary feasibility reports for health and family planning projects; a team to evaluate the malaria project; and a consultant to assess the feasibility of a proposed epidemiological survey. Most of USAID's long-term advisors are hired through independent private consulting firms or universities based in the United States. In recent years, an increasing amount of AID's assistance has been funneled through consulting groups, and many firms have been created in response to this policy.

The competition for AID contracts is intense. The lengthy selection process begins when AID's country health office sends out a request for proposals from interested consulting groups describing how the job will be done.[4] The proposals undergo competitive review, and the winning group is selected to work in the country under the supervision of the local AID office. Because of this process, the immediate focus of the consulting groups is often on obtaining the contract and meeting AID's requirements, while the realities of the recipient country's health needs may fall into the background. By hiring a consulting firm that provides a group of consultants as part of a package, AID avoids the time-consuming process of hiring individual consultants one by one. Both staff members in the AID Nepal country office and Nepali officials observed, however, that some advisors in the consulting package are not always technically appropriate to the needs of the project.

The consultant system also serves to lighten the weight of AID's presence in the recipient country, at least from the American point of view. According to AID policy, AID's role is to assist and advise but not to take command of projects. An AID director explained that by using consultants to work on projects with the government, AID is able to manage assistance to programs from a distance, keeping its own role less visible. Frequently, AID officers mentioned their efforts to minimize the visibility of their own direct participation and influence in government projects. Several AID advisors in Nepal described their attempt to attribute all collaborative work to their Nepali counterparts. However, Nepalis always referred to all AID employees, both staff members and contracted advisors, as AID personnel.

USAID's stated goal for health in Nepal for 1975–80 was to strengthen and expand ICHP through financial and technical assistance. Technical assistance took the form of long-term advisors and short-term consultants provided by Health Associates, a private consulting firm in New York. (Health Associates is a pseudonym for this contracting group.) Health Associates' basic team of four long-term advisors worked with ICHP for five years, from 1977 to 1981. The "chief of party," or head of the team, was a physician. He helped ICHP develop and test management systems, survey designs, and program evaluations for basic health services. He also coordinated USAID's short-term consultant contracts and other assistance to the program. The second advisor was an operational research analyst who worked with the Health Planning Unit as a management system analyst. The third, a management training specialist, helped ICHP train supervisory staff in field management and assisted in implementation and evaluation. The fourth advisor, an expert in educational planning, served as a training specialist, designing curriculum and developing teaching methods for training health workers in integrated community health care.

Interaction Between the Government and the Agencies

Linkages between the Nepali health bureaucracy and the donor agencies are complicated and do not always provide for an adequate flow of information. For example, at WHO's policy level, Nepal participates in policy formulation by sending representatives to meetings in Geneva. These representatives usually include very senior members of the health bureaucracy, such as the Minister and Secretary of Health. Other representatives may be selected for a variety of reasons, which may not always reflect their qualifications. In any case, representatives are not likely to be familiar with rural health resources and conditions, since they are usually Western-educated members of elite families in Kathmandu.

Based on these meetings, WHO assumes that it has government commitment to the policy decisions that are made. But at the next level, health policy encounters a gap in the Nepali system between the Palace Secretariat, Nepal's policy making body, and the Central Secretariat, which is responsible for implementation. Thus, consultants and advisors from WHO, USAID, and other agencies arrive in Nepal to assist in carrying out policies, but the Nepalis they work with in the Ministry of Health are not the ones who made policy commitments in Nepal or Geneva. In general, foreigners in Nepal have very little contact with the Palace Secretariat.

Within the agencies, the common practice of hiring consultants to carry out programs creates another gap. The policies are handed down for translation into programs by agency staff, who then hire consultants to work with Nepali officials. The consultants are outsiders who have not participated in the policymaking process. Although technically competent, they often know little about the agencies' policies and administrative procedures or about the Nepali system. Thus, at the implementation level, neither consultants representing the agencies nor most Nepali officials in the ministry have direct links to policymaking or a comprehensive view of the policies and programs.

Using USAID as an example, Figure 2 shows how interaction between the government and the donor agencies is concentrated at the planning and upper implementation levels. Although a few foreign advisors worked full-time in the field, implementation of ICHP at the local level was left almost entirely to the government. Advisors from both USAID and WHO had some contact with ICHP supervisory staff and made occasional field visits, but most contact took place with Nepali officials in Kathmandu. Thus, foreign advisors had little experience with either the highest levels of the Nepal government or with the district and village administration—and little access to information about conditions in rural Nepal.

Of course, many other donors contributed in a variety of ways to ICHP, although none were as directly involved in shaping policy and plans as WHO and USAID. The Canadian International Development Agency provided the only

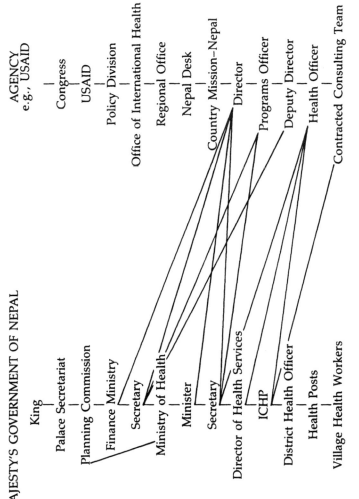

HIS MAJESTY'S GOVERNMENT OF NEPAL

King

Palace Secretariat

Planning Commission

Finance Ministry

Secretary

Ministry of Health

Minister

Secretary

Director of Health Services

ICHP

District Health Officer

Health Posts

Village Health Workers

AGENCY
e.g., USAID

Congress

USAID

Policy Division

Office of International Health

Regional Office

Nepal Desk

Country Mission–Nepal

Director

Programs Officer

Deputy Director

Health Officer

Contracted Consulting Team

FIGURE 2 *Contact Points Between the Nepal Government and the International Health Agencies*

other full-time consultant to an ICHP-related activity, a nurse associated with the Institute of Medicine. Often, several donors were involved in different aspects of the same area, such as training. Canada's assistance to the training of health workers who would be assigned to ICHP included the building of two training schools (in Surkhet and Dhankuta), building health posts in the surrounding area to serve as field training centers, and developing curriculum at the Institute of Medicine (IOM). The Institute of Medicine in Kathmandu trained all categories of health workers in the health structure, including those in ICHP. Two USAID short-term consultants also assisted with curriculum development at the Institute of Medicine. The United Nations Fund for Population Activities gave assistance mainly for in-service training of health workers, conducted by the Department of Health Services.

Foreign assistance to the construction of health training schools illustrates the dilemma that aid agencies often face when their desire to minimize their visibility conflicts with the bureaucratic value of accountability. The Canadians played a highly visible role in constructing the schools in Surkhet and Dhankuta. They maintained control by importing Canadian engineers and personnel to supervise the project, with Nepalis hired as contractors and construction workers. USAID chose to play a less visible role by giving the Institute of Medicine funds to supervise construction, hire workers, and so on for the schools in Pokhara and Birganj. In 1979, AID officials were having difficulty accounting for these funds because the Institute had so far produced no material results. Donors who find themselves in this awkward position often become more involved in carrying out projects than they might ideally want to be.

The presence of several donors often intensifies competition among them to find outlets for their funds. These outlets are limited because a government receiving aid must spend administrative time and energy dealing with donors, managing programs into which aid is funneled, and accounting for monies spent. Thus, only a limited amount of assistance can be absorbed by a given program, according to the capacity of its administrative structure. Governments in developing countries such as Nepal are under constant pressure to accept assistance, however, because of complex international political and economic issues surrounding foreign aid, and because donor agencies thrive on giving assistance. The agencies must continue funding programs to maintain their large bureaucracies, which are staffed with career officers who must maintain a role in the organization to ensure their own future.

When smallpox was at last eradicated, for example, new jobs had to be found for the domestic and international workers who had been employed in smallpox eradication programs. This meant finding new projects. In Nepal, the replacement was the Expanded Program of Immunization (EPI), which was developed by UNICEF and WHO as a new vertical program rather than as an integral part of ICHP, even though the official policy of both agencies supported integration. The rationalization given by the agencies for developing EPI as a separate project was the high-priority need to immunize infants and pregnant women, at a time when ICHP had limited resources for undertaking the proposed project. Not only do the many donors currently in Nepal compete to maintain their role, but newcomers frequently pressure the government to accept their assistance as well.

Competition among donors affected Nepal's programs in family planning and in maternal and child health. UNICEF's activity centered on maternal and child health, whereas USAID emphasized direct family planning. Representatives of the two agencies were at odds over what constituted maternal and child health activities, and the Nepal government was caught between them. Both agencies gave assistance for family planning and maternal and child health to the vertical Family Planning Program and to ICHP. Such situations could possibly be avoided if the agencies assisted programs defined by the Nepal government, and not by the agencies. However, the government may inadvertently encourage competition among donors by not always providing clearly defined policies, programs, and requests for assistance.

The construction of a large teaching hospital in Kathmandu is another example of competition among donors. The government wanted a 500-bed hospital, but the major aid agencies were not supporting the proposal because they believed that it would siphon resources away from the rural health services. As a compromise, the agencies agreed to support a training program at the Institute of Medicine that would prepare doctors to work in rural areas, and to help fund small teaching hospitals in districts in order to meet the acute need for doctors at the district level. But the government still wanted the large hospital in Kathmandu, and because of the competitive funding environment it was able to negotiate successfully for the hospital. Eventually, Japan, a new donor in the health field, provided the funds.

Health post construction illustrates the confusion that results from too many donors and too little coordination. Health posts were a high priority in Nepal. As one advisor said, the government had to take all the assistance that came along in order for health post construction to meet its target of 800 health posts by 1985, despite the shortage of trained health workers to staff the posts. Given this encouragement, most donors allocated funds for the purpose: the Netherlands, Britain, Japan, Canada, West Germany, the United States, Switzerland, and the World Bank all contributed. Some donors simply gave money for building, but others became directly involved in the construction, using their own criteria for building design, materials, and contracting arrangements. For example, the Swiss development agency supported a number of existing health posts and was building new ones in the Hill Development Project in Jiri, which it was funding. The Swiss director said that these health posts were run according to Nepal government guidelines, but that Swiss aid had its own specifications for such areas as roofing materials and window size which did not always match specifications used by the government and other donors.

Donors' reports on projects typically state that villagers' expectations and needs are taken into consideration, but it is not clear how these are assessed or accommodated. Buildings are often modeled on foreign designs that have been used in other Third World countries, without taking into consideration either the local climate or local resources. Cement is in extremely short supply in Nepal, and it is difficult to transport into many hill areas. When local panchayats constructed a mud-and-stone health post with their own resources and labor, the government often built a *pukka* (cement) health post in the same area to replace it, saying that the new one met the Department of Health Services' specifications, which in turn were based on foreign advice. This chain of events discouraged local initiative. Villagers said they would prefer that the government use its resources to meet other needs rather than duplicate their own efforts just to meet foreign specifications and Nepali political pressures. Thus, local priorities may be submerged under the complex interactions among the government and the agencies, each with its own priorities and approach.

Nepali Administrators and International Advisors

Daily working relationships between Nepali administrators and international advisors reflected cultural differences between the Nepali and agency bureaucracies.

USAID's contract advisors from Health Associates were the foreigners most directly involved with ICHP. They worked with assigned Nepali counterparts—planners and administrators—in the Department of Health Services, where each advisor had a desk. In fact, the little building that had been partitioned into offices for ICHP had desks for three Health Associates advisors and two WHO consultants in 1978–79. On entering it, one was struck by the high proportion of foreign advisors and by the long line of foreigners usually waiting to see the ICHP chief. Health Associates and WHO advisors to Nepal's Health Planning Unit similarly had desks in the Planning Unit office.

Since the ICHP building was cramped and poorly equipped, Health Associates also rented a separate office building in the Ministry of Health complex. There they had more of the amenities of Western offices, such as a telephone, office equipment, reproduction materials, supplies, a library, bathroom facilities, and space for clerical assistance and for the two jeep drivers. They could also stay in closer contact with USAID and have a place to work when government offices were closed for the frequent Nepali holidays. Similarly, WHO provided its advisors with second offices in the WHO building because of the limited space and support services available in government offices.

During the workday, Health Associates advisors frequently worked in their own office building, since their Nepali counterparts were often not available—being either on leave or seconded to other duties—and from a pragmatic perspective, more could be accomplished in these better-equipped and more spacious surroundings. Also, some advisors were sensitive to the possibility that their presence might be an intrusion in the Nepali offices. Although Nepalis, especially the training officers, went to the Health Associates office, the separate office building for consultants tended to isolate them from Nepali officials and encouraged them to interact more with other foreigners. Creating offices that mirrored the consultants' own bureaucratic culture was common practice among donor agencies. Thus, they maintained a certain cultural distance, even while working in Nepal.

As part of my effort to find out how foreign donors obtained and exchanged information with Nepali officials and other foreigners, I asked Nepali counterparts to describe and diagram their perception of the foreign advisors' relationship to ICHP. Their responses varied. A planning officer at the Ministry of Health described the advisors as technicians and diagramed them as separate units without connecting lines to either their counterparts or assigned offices. A Nepali medical officer in ICHP diagramed the relationship by using arrows connecting advisors to their counterparts, showing that the Health Associates advisor for supervision related to the ICHP officer in charge of field supervision; the advisor on training related to the training officer; the senior medical advisor and chief of the Health Associates team related directly to the ICHP chief; the WHO advisor for immunization worked directly with the ICHP chief; and so on.

The advisors' perceptions of their own roles varied as well. The senior Health Associates advisor was concerned about his level of involvement. He said that he had become more involved in planning and implementation than he desired because he had stepped in when Nepali officials were not available. At that time, he alone knew the ICHP budget in detail. He said that ICHP staff considered advisors useful because advisors had efficient typists, printing facilities, budgets, and staff, which enabled them to get things done. If the Nepalis had these same resources, he added, they could do as much.

One WHO advisor saw *no* effective role for himself or other advisors in ICHP. He thought that the Nepalis saw advisors as a necessary encumbrance, as part of the aid package, and rarely put them to work. Often, no Nepali counterparts were assigned to advisors, or they existed in name only. The WHO advisor said that he might be asked to do a specific project, such as write a report or find an overseas fellowship, but that basically advisors had to initiate or create their own niche, which sometimes meant starting a new program.

Another foreign advisor, although frustrated by his lack of direct access to senior health officials, did not worry as much as others about his immediate relationships and the outcomes of the program. He saw his role to be that of developing a system—establishing a process—and not delivering health services. This perception differed little, in his opinion, from the government's objectives, which he described as first, politics; next, employment; and last, health. Several Nepali officials who worked with this advisor commented that although he worked hard, his background, training, and approach to health planning were inappropriate for Nepal's resources and stage of development. One Nepali counterpart summarized these comments by saying, "He is the wrong man, in the wrong place, at the wrong time."

The Secretary of Health's perception of consultants agreed with that of the WHO advisor: consultants were part of the aid package. The ICHP chief thought that advisors were useful for filling gaps but that they were too abundant. Although he was trying to cut back the number, it was hard to persuade donors not to replace them. For example, although the WHO medical advisor to ICHP was being cut out, he would be replaced by an operation officer for supervision.

Other Nepalis I interviewed described the flood of foreign advisors and representatives as one of the "penalties" of aid. One senior health official commented, ' There are so many foreigners, who each come with schemes which just create more work for the government. The government is now trying to limit the number of small donors, but we have commitments to those already here, so nothing can be done about these." Many foreigners were accustomed to working with colleagues and therefore expected to have Nepali counterparts, although often these did not materialize. Agencies had unrealistic ideas about Nepali staffing potential and created a need for national counterparts which the government could not meet.

Nepalis commented on the many types, qualities, and abilities of advisors, but they questioned the high cost even for those whom they considered most helpful. For a foreign staff member or advisor in Nepal, the United Nations Development Program budgets $75,000 per year, or 1 million rupees, excluding agency overhead.* By contrast, the official cost to the government for a Nepali officer is between 20,000 and 30,000 rupees per year, yielding a ratio of one foreigner for every thirty to fifty Nepali counterparts (Shrestha 1983:1).

In 1978–79, Nepalis frequently referred to ICHP as a USAID or WHO program (or as the program of a specific USAID advisor, i.e., Dr. X's program), thus clearly identifying it as foreign. This perception reveals much about the advisors' role, for despite their sensitivity about visibility, the advisors were highly visible in all aspects of the program and appeared to have the most invested in its success. And in fact, a look at the typical life-style and career patterns in the foreign aid community reveals that in some ways the foreign advisors did stand to gain more personal and professional benefits from a program's success than their Nepali counterparts.

In 1979 more than 700 foreigners were working with do-

---

*In 1978, one U.S. dollar equaled approximately eleven Nepali rupees.

nor aid programs and the diplomatic corps in Kathmandu. The United Nations and its specialized agencies had 118 representatives and long-term consultants there. To this figure must be added those working with the eighteen bilateral aid organizations (estimated at 355, without short-term consultants), religious missions, and voluntary organizations, as well as the diplomatic corps, serving twenty embassies in Nepal and staffed by an estimated 260 foreigners (Thapa 1981). Many were involved with health-related activities.

Foreign advisors varied as to nationality, personal background, and professional experience, but usually they were Westerners. Most advisors to ICHP or related health projects were from Europe or North America, and, except for a Canadian administrator/nurse, and English nurse-midwife educator, and an American administrator, all were male. Religious missions and private health organizations (such as the Dooley Foundation, Save the Children, and Britain Nepal Medical Trust) had female doctors and nurses, mostly in direct clinical service or teaching, although some were administrators.

Although foreigners live in various parts of Kathmandu, they tend to cluster in certain areas where enterprising Nepalis have built new houses with Western-style amenities and plumbing, specifically for the purpose of renting to foreigners. These houses are well equipped and spacious by most Western standards, many being located in large gardens surrounded by trees and greenery. Some organizations, such as USAID and the Canadian International Development Agency, furnish them with imported appliances and Western-style furniture made by local craftsmen. Allowances are provided for domestic servants—cooks, bearers, watchmen, gardeners, and ayahs (nannies). Utilities are often maintained and paid for by the donor organization.

In addition, donor agencies offset the drawbacks of living abroad by offering high salaries (many of them tax-exempt, which often enable consultants to accumulate large savings); paying school fees; providing cars, often with chauffeurs; and arranging for access to commissary or duty-free provisions. The agencies also provide high pensions. One advisor, who had worked with WHO for four years, said that he was frustrated with his professional responsibilities, but, nevertheless, had requested a one-year extension to his contract in order to be eligible for the excellent pension scheme offered to United Nations employees after five years of service. If as Stiller and Yadev (1979:58) have observed, foreign aid is good business for Kathmandu, it is equally profitable for foreign advisors, many of whom live at a social and economic level above what they could expect in their home country.

Thus, in addition to humanitarian and professional motives, financial motives cannot be overlooked as a reason for accepting foreign consultancies. Hall and Dieffenback (1973) have questioned whether such inflated salaries and lifestyles do not interfere with fulfilling job responsibilities and achieving development goals. They certainly increase the gulf between the advisors and their Nepali counterparts, who usually earn only a small fraction (one-tenth to one-twentieth) of an advisor's salary. As a practical matter, the unequal provision for per diem expenses (in 1979, 18 rupees per day for government officials and approximately 200 rupees per day for USAID advisors) complicates the working relationship between advisors and their Nepali counterparts and serves to discourage joint field travel.

Many advisors also enjoy higher status and greater power than they would at home. Consultants and advisors are called "experts" in their areas of technical specialization and are often placed in positions in which they can design large-scale projects. Merely because they are foreigners, they can often bypass their Nepali counterparts who have similar training and positions. In Nepal, as in India and other developing countries, foreign advisors frequently meet with senior government officials, including the minister and secretary of health, senior officers in related ministries, and members of the Planning Commission, as well as with prominent Kathmandu residents, for professional purposes and at official social events. Most would not have such access to powerful decision makers in their home universities, health departments, or governments, or even within the donor organizations that employ them.

Some advisors with specialized technical training appeared frustrated at being placed in positions that made inadequate use of special abilities. In many areas, Nepali resources are not adequate to take advantage of specialized knowledge. But despite personal inconvenience and professional frustration, advisors are reluctant to give up the attractions, secondary gains, and security associated with membership in the international aid community.

All of the foreign advisors to ICHP had had previous overseas experience as advisors. Some said they wanted to return home to work after completing their assignments in Nepal, but all were later reported to have taken assignments with donor agencies in other countries. Transfer to another country or agency is usually accompanied by a promotion and more benefits. The longer the overseas experience, the harder it is to reenter employment at home. Thus, membership in the foreign aid community becomes a way of life.

Social exchanges are frequent among many of the advisors, who naturally turn to each other for companionship; but many find it difficult to mix informally with Nepalis. Although advisors frequently meet high-level Nepalis in professional and formal settings, they do not typically socialize with them at a more personal, informal level. Even wealthy Nepalis, with their traditional homes and cuisine, may feel at a disadvantage if they socialize with foreigners who have luxurious homes and serve imported food and liquor. Most foreigners, therefore, serve as their own reference group, remaining socially and culturally apart from the people they aim to serve.

This social and cultural distance from the Nepalis permeates professional life as well. Foreign advisors who deal with the Nepali bureaucracy face an administrative system that superficially resembles Western bureaucracies but actually functions on the basis of familial, patron-client, caste, regional, and ethnic loyalties. Not understanding this, advisors assess Nepali counterparts using Western bureaucratic standards, in which an employee is supposed to be judged not by who he is but by his job performance; by the impression he makes on his superiors; and by his conformity to certain standards of dress, language, and behavior. As a result, foreign advisors often function in an environment of misunderstanding, confusion, and frustration.

Advisors have little opportunity, in any event, to learn about the local system. They are usually posted to a country mission for two to four years to carry out specific projects of limited duration. Their actual stay typically is foreshortened, since the first months are preoccupied with "settling-in"—adjusting to a new social and work environment—and the last months with transfer and moving arrangements, "settling-out." Advisors therefore have little time to establish more than formal work relationships with government officials. Neither donor agencies nor government officials recognize a need for cultural orientation, and so most advisors do not receive language training or any other form of cultural preparation as part of their official briefings.

Although there is a notion that advisors could do a better job by getting to know Nepal and their Nepali colleagues, the administrative demands of donor agencies, geared to their headquarters' procedures and needs, are often so great that advisors must spend much of their time in the agency office. The fact that the colleagues and superiors who control advancement are also located at headquarters strengthens office ties. One Nepali official wrote, "Since most [advisors] are employed by donor agencies, they are always beholden to the wishes of their supervisors in capitals other than Kathmandu, and the busiest days of those [advisors] are when their bosses visit Nepal" (Shrestha 1983:224). Agency administrators may note that a particular advisor gets along well with Nepalis, but this quality is rarely given as a reason for promotion. The typical advisor's relationship with Nepali colleagues is commonly single stranded, job related, and impersonal.

The situation is much more complex for the Nepali bureaucrat. He is judged not only on training and on job performance but also on personal affiliation. Familial and interpersonal relationships are critically important in determining the course of his career. Relationships within the bureaucracy are multistranded, personal, and long-term, sometimes extending over generations. A person's relationship to his superiors is therefore determined not only by formal lines of authority but also by kinship and caste. Nepalis who are removed from the Kathmandu central elite, both by kinship and by geographical distance, use the term "source and force" repeatedly in explaining their undesirable situation. Having "source and force" means "having a contact (friend or relative) who has the power to do what you want him to do." Since jobs are scarce—especially good ones in desirable locations—competition and insecurity are intense. Even senior Nepali officials believe that their competitors also have "source": "The ultimate belief is that every rule, every law and every structure could be bent to one's purpose if an adequate 'source' were at hand" (Stiller and Yadav 1979:120).

Nepali bureaucrats also have developed a tradition of avoiding direct personal responsibility for administrative action and policy recommendations. Since the Nepal government structure vests policymaking power principally in the king and the Palace Secretariat, officials in the ministries are in the position of implementing policies over which they have little control. Yet if a program is not successful, blame may be placed on the implementors rather than on those who formulated policy. As a result, Nepalis tend to share responsibility among several officials, so that no one person can be blamed if things go wrong. This way of spreading responsibility for carrying out Palace-designed programs also extends to internationally designed and assisted programs such as ICHP (Rose 1982:35).

The typical Nepali administrator cannot afford to take a stand in opposition to government policy, to his supervisor, or to family members that would single him out for reproach. To displease those in power might result in transfer to a less desirable post in which one would have less influence. Nepalis often comment, for example, that someone must have done something wrong to have been appointed chief of the Indent and Procurement Section of the Department of Health Services, defined as a "punishment post." The person punished in this way must use "source and force" to obtain transfer to a more desirable post until he is restored to favor. This strategy requires being close to those in power at the center; thus, health workers are reluctant to accept district assignments, especially in remote areas. Those who must work in rural areas often spend considerable time away from their rural post to make the desired contacts in Kathmandu.

Foreign advisors and Nepali administrators have different perceptions of their roles that affect their approaches to their work. Many advisors define their role as providing solutions to problems. To them, the completion of a health plan or the construction of a health post means that they have successfully completed their assignment. They will be judged according to what they were able to accomplish and their ability to demonstrate results for money spent. Nepali officials do not share this orientation. Instead, they see themselves as acting in an environment where the bureaucrat cannot usually afford to take initiative and distinguish himself. He must be attuned to his superior's personal goals and to his own position and family needs, which are the criteria by which he will be judged. Aid projects provide jobs with special benefits, which end when the project is completed or withdrawn. Knowing that individual consultants and project schemes come and go in a relatively short time, a Nepali may agree to a program that he knows is inappropriate for Nepal in order to ensure his own job security. For the Nepali, personal success depends less on the short-term success of a particular program than on the long-term art of personal diplomacy. For the foreign advisor, personal success—the extension of his job, career advancement, and higher status in the foreign aid community—depends more on successful programs (although an advisor of course cannot afford to displease *his* home agency either).

Nepali bureaucrats probably understand Western bureaucracies better than Westerners understand the Nepali bureaucracy. Advisors sense the differences in values and modes of operation, but their comments show that they do not really understand the differences or how they affect the way things work. Advisors know that the Nepalis exchange information through personal contacts and not through the official channels, but many do not understand the kin and personal connections among those they see clustered in offices before the workday begins or in informal settings after work, nor do they understand how these people are connected to those in power. Even when foreigners do understand the informal Nepali networks, they can never gain access to them. Foreign advisors frequently mentioned to me that they would like to know more about the culture of the Nepali bureaucracy to help them identify decision makers and understand the decision-making process. In my view, foreigners find it difficult to understand the cues and signs in Kathmandu and almost impossible to interpret the complex network of relationships in district and local administration—an essential aspect of understanding how rural health programs are implemented and how they are interpreted at each level of the Nepali system. Thus, the effort to deliver health services to rural Nepal encountered not only structural barriers to communication within the Nepali and Western bureaucracies but cultural barriers as well.

3

Policies and Plans

In the realm of international health aid, donor agencies exert a strong influence over the policies of many recipient governments. Certainly their influence has been strong in Nepal. To understand the decisions that created Nepal's rural health program, one must first look at the trends in policy among international health agencies and in Western scientific health thinking as a whole, as they have developed in recent decades. It is a history that progresses from early efforts to control epidemics to the modern emphasis on providing rural health services and preventive care.

The nineteenth-century colonial powers entered the field of international health to protect their nationals in the colonial service and, by extension, their own nations from communicable disease epidemics. The quarantine movement of the period developed from this motive, and quarantinable diseases were the main concern of the first international health organizations, the Pan American Sanitary Bureau (1902) and L'Office Internationale d'Hygiene Publique (1909). The League of Nations Health Office assumed responsibility for international quarantine in 1923, which in turn was undertaken by the World Health Organization in 1948 (Brockquarantine to the control and eradication of epidemic diseases such as smallpox and malaria at their source (Taylor 1979:803).

Physicians imported to provide care for colonial service employees, for plantation owners and workers, and for others involved in trade brought modern medical care to some Third World countries. Religious missions, which combined medical work with religious goals, were responsible for introducing allopathic medicine into many others. Their early efforts concentrated on curative work, hospitals, and training programs (Taylor 1975:805). In some developing countries (for example, Tanzania and Malawi), mission-supported medical programs and institutions accounted for more than 40 percent of all professional allopathic health care as recently as 1968 (Bryant 1969:304). Recently, directors of mission projects have sought closer relationships with government programs and have begun to emphasize preventive medicine.

Following World War II, as the colonial period ended and new independent nations emerged throughout the Third World, large-scale economic assistance from "developed" countries to "developing" or Third World countries became an important part of international diplomacy. On the premise that "the developed world possessed both the talent and capital for helping backward countries to develop" (Tendler 1976:10), assistance was given for reasons that ranged from humanitarian to economic, political, and military concerns. The primary objective of most foreign aid appears to have been either political or economic: for example, foreign aid was intended to ensure a continuing supply of cheap natural resources (e.g., bauxite) and agricultural goods, and to develop markets for the finished products of industrialized nations.

Whereas early programs emphasized aid for agriculture and industry, today the diversity and scale of assistance are enormous. Since international planners now see health problems as an obstacle to development, most developing countries receive foreign aid for health and population programs as well as to assist economic development both directly and indirectly. By 1977 the estimated volume of external assistance for health services to all countries was substantial—

about $400 million annually. If the definition of health services is expanded to include family planning, water supply, sanitation, and nutrition, external assistance for health to all countries in 1977 totaled approximately $1.1 billion (World Bank 1978:23).

The donors of international health aid included multilateral agencies, such as WHO; bilateral agencies, such as USAID; and private organizations, such as foundations, voluntary groups, and religious missions. Along with their funds came policy guidelines and programmatic influences. The international donor agencies, on the strength of their economic resources, have thus dominated health policy and practices in the Third World since World War II—"He who pays the piper, calls the tune."

International Health Policy and Nepal

Hospital-Based and Vertical Programs

From the 1940s to the 1960s, international policies followed two paths: 1) hospital care and medical and nursing education, and 2) public health programs to prevent or control communicable diseases. Funding for the first went to medical and nursing schools, large teaching hospitals, and maternal and child health care units (World Bank 1979:23). This policy created hospital systems that were based in urban areas, with sophisticated technology and highly trained personnel that were primarily accessible to small, elite sections of the population (Djukanovic and Mach 1975:7). Around the world, disease-specific programs—referred to as vertical or categorical programs—were organized to control such infectious diseases as smallpox, leprosy, tuberculosis, malaria, and yaws at the community level. The vertical programs usually had a semiautonomous status within the government, were administered and supervised by special personnel, and trained paramedical workers for a single purpose. The short-term perspective of these programs was a key element, for they were designed to train and employ temporary, independent staff whose jobs would end after a few years, when the task was done.

In Asia the campaign to eradicate malaria, which was identified as one of the major health-related obstacles to development in the 1950s, was planned mainly by WHO and USAID. This program, which was the entry point of large-scale health assistance in Nepal, illustrates the impact that foreign assistance can have in recipient countries. Although Nepal was not affected as directly by the initial stages of international assistance as its more accessible neighbors, the development of international health programs there since 1951 has followed the pattern established in other countries.

Malaria was a serious problem in Nepal especially in the Terai, where it made much of the country's richest farmland inaccessible. USAID helped finance and start a countrywide eradication program in 1954. At the same time, WHO started a pilot/demonstration program in the Rapti Valley, where six WHO advisors trained Nepali workers and supervised eradication measures. The Nepal government, having acquired some expertise, expanded the program in 1958. In each case the accepted strategy was to eradicate malaria by eliminating the mosquitoes that transmit the malaria parasite to man. This was to be achieved by large-scale spraying with DDT and by destroying mosquito habitats. In addition to an all-out attack on mosquitoes, large populations of Nepalis were given chloraquine as a prophylactic treatment to prevent malaria.

Campaigns such as these, backed by sufficient resources and international cooperation, sharply reduced the incidence of malaria in almost all countries where they were carried out (Voulgaropoulos 1977:36). In Nepal, the malaria eradication program was the largest and most successful health program of its time. Workers were well trained to complete clearly defined tasks; the program was well supervised, managed, and administered; and almost 50 percent of the population in malarial areas received services.

By the late 1960s, however, as the threat of malaria eased in many countries, foreign donors began to withdraw assistance from malaria eradication programs. Although malaria had been controlled, the number of cases having fallen sharply, it had not been eradicated. Recipient governments, including that of Nepal, which had depended on the technology and resources provided by the donor agencies, were unable to maintain the programs at adequate levels on their own. As a result of diminished foreign aid and the rise of the Anopheles mosquito's resistance to DDT, the incidence of malaria began to rise again.

Other vertical programs in Nepal were the Leprosy and Tuberculosis Control Project, launched in 1964/1965; the Smallpox Eradication Project, launched in 1967/1968, which eradicated smallpox in the 1970s; and the Family Planning and Child Welfare Project, begun in 1968. (See Appendix 1: A Chronology of Health-Sector Events in Nepal.)

The Family Planning Project was the result of another major policy trend that surfaced during the late 1960s. Donor agencies were turning their attention at this time to rapid population growth, which they viewed as a major health-related problem impeding modernization and economic development. As worldwide infant mortality rates gradually fell because of disease control programs and improved nutrition and sanitation, as well as broader social and economic developments, population rates began to rise rapidly after World War II. It was not until the mid-1960s, however, that family planning programs began to be supported. As most agencies began financing population-related programs, aid for this purpose mounted impressively. In 1965, USAID's worldwide budget for family planning was $1.9 million, or about 5.5 percent of its total budget for health and population programs; in 1978 its budget for family planning was $177 million, or 59.4 percent of the total.[1] This money supported family planning and the provision of birth control techniques, training for personnel, and the creation of new high-level institutions (such as population commissions and family planning coordination boards) in countries reluctant to undertake population-related programs within existing structures.

Family planning assistance, despite its scale, has had only limited success in reducing the rate of population growth in most countries. The evidence suggests that social and cultural factors have had much to do with the lack of results.

Policymakers overlooked the cultural context of childbearing (Mamdani 1972), and indications are that decreases in population growth are linked not only to family planning programs but more significantly to social, economic, and political changes (Ratcliffe 1978), including higher literacy rates, improved status of women, improved access to health and education services, lower unemployment, and income leveling (Rifkin 1977:33).

As of 1976, Nepal's rate of population growth remained high—over 2.5 percent per year. Nepali women traditionally marry early and continue having children throughout their fertile years. Because sons are strongly preferred, couples have many children, an average of 6.8 per married woman (UNICEF 1982:25), in the hope that at least one or two sons will survive until adulthood. Few couples know about or have access to modern means of contraception, despite government attempts to promote family planning.

In response to the discouraging results of the family planning programs, international health policy has changed direction again. Donor agencies now favor incorporating family planning services into broader health and rural development programs, including agricultural, educational, and private sector projects.

The Shift to Integrated Basic Health Services

Along with the emphasis on family planning, another extremely important policy shift was occurring during the 1960s. The donor agencies recognized that their previous hospital-based approach typically delivered services only to urban areas, where only a small portion of the population lived. Such disease-specific or vertical programs, though sometimes successful, were expensive to operate and were taking longer to complete than initially planned. Moreover, they failed to address the underlying causes of poor health, such as poor nutrition, polluted water, inadequate preventive care, poor hygiene, and so on. The response to these shortcomings was an entirely new approach, the concept of basic health services, which was developed in the 1960s and 1970s by the donor agencies under the leadership of UNICEF and WHO.

This new approach was allied with a general shift among international aid agencies to rural development. In 1973, for example, the U.S. Congress mandated foreign assistance for low-cost public health programs that would reach the majority of the rural poor in the countries served. Foreign assistance moved away from aiding large infrastructural and urban-based projects, such as hospitals and medical schools (Cochrane 1980; Hoben 1980:356), to constructing, equipping, and staffing rural health centers and health posts; providing technical assistance for training new categories of health workers; and assisting with some of the operating costs of health institutions.

Basic health services were defined as providing immunization; assistance to mothers during pregnancy and delivery; postnatal and child care; appropriate contraceptive advice in countries accepting family planning policies; adequate, safe, and accessible water supplies; sanitation and vector control; health and nutrition education; diagnosis and treatment for simple diseases; first aid and emergency treatment; and facilities for referral. These services would be offered by a system of district hospitals and rural health posts.

One of the major innovations of this approach was "integration," in which the single-purpose health workers in the vertical health programs (such as those for smallpox and malaria) were to be converted into multipurpose health workers. These multipurpose workers would combine the work of several vertical workers; for example, they would detect malaria and leprosy cases as well as provide simple health care, preventive care, and health education. Through short retraining courses, vertical program workers could learn to be "generalists," and thus the manpower available for integrated health services would grow rapidly. Integration would deliver preventive, promotive, and curative services through a single administrative structure. It was expected to reduce overhead and service delivery costs, thus providing a cost-effective way to extend health and family planning services to rural areas.

In accordance with the new emphasis on rural development, and in an attempt to combine several vertical health programs, the integrated basic health approach was introduced in Nepal in the late 1960s and dominated health policy and planning there in the 1970s.

The integrated approach in Nepal, which was promoted through assistance mainly from WHO, USAID, and UNICEF, reflected attempts by these agencies to integrate administratively their own departments of health, population, and nutrition. It also coincided with the Nepal government's stated policy of spreading social benefits to all parts of the nation, which was expressed in the fourth five-year development plan (for 1970–75). According to a pronouncement by the king, the government sought to provide at least minimum health services to the maximum possible number of people, especially the rural majority. The government formalized this commitment by creating the Division of Integrated Basic Health Services (IBHS) within the Department of Health Services in 1971.

Still another motive was at work. Because the incidence of malaria had decreased, and USAID and other international donors were ready to withdraw their support from malaria eradication programs, hundreds of health workers and administrators in Nepal, as well as international malaria specialists, would soon be unemployed if other programs were not developed to absorb them. The Integrated Basic Health Services helped provide a solution.

The Integrated Basic Health Services was designed to expand health and family planning services, especially to rural areas, using the Nepal Malaria Eradication Program's well-organized infrastructure and trained cadre of workers. In mid-1973 the Nepal government, WHO, and USAID jointly started two pilot projects to test two strategies for integration—that is, for replacing the single-purpose malaria field worker with a multipurpose health and family planning worker. The donor agencies also wanted to evaluate the effectiveness of integrating family planning services with other health services—a prospect that was arousing international controversy among population and public health experts at the time. In addition, they hoped to demonstrate a more effective program for slowing Nepal's rapid population growth.

The pilot projects were designed and funded primarily by the international donor agencies, which also made available extensive advisory and supervisory services during an eighteen-month period. They were started in two districts, with a total of fourteen health posts covering a population of about 300,000. Kaski District, in the western hills, and Bara District, in the southern Terai plains, were selected as being representative of the geographic, communication, logistic, administrative, and transportation difficulties typically encountered in the country.

The key differences between the projects lay in their administrative structures. In Kaski District, with three health posts, the malaria organization was retained. No changes were made in staff and funding or in the geographic and population jurisdiction assigned to the workers, but other functions were added. This policy decision was made to determine whether malaria workers could perform the additional tasks of checking for diseases other than malaria and providing family planning information during house visits.

In Bara District, with eleven health posts, a new system was created, representing a much more dramatic departure from the old malaria program. Here, responsibility for directing, supervising, and coordinating the integrated program was given to the newly established Division of Integrated Basic Health Services. In theory, the Kathmandu central office of Integrated Basic Health Services worked through the Zonal Health Office and Hospital, which served as the referral institution for the District Hospital and Health Office, which in turn was the referral institution for the eleven health posts in Bara. Each health post served a population of about 25,000, which included ten to twelve village panchayats. The health post area was divided into three to seven *veks,* or localities, each with an average population of 5,000 and each the responsibility of a single junior auxiliary health worker, later called a village health worker (Nepal/ Berkeley 1975:235). The village health worker (VHW) was a villager with six weeks of basic health training whose main responsibility was to provide preventive care and health education through home visits in his own locality.

Each VHW was attached to a health post. The health posts were planned to provide ambulatory medical care, including treatment and follow-up of tuberculosis and leprosy cases; family planning services, including education and treatment for contraceptive complications; periodic sterilization camps; and maternal and child health services, including deliveries of babies, antenatal and postnatal care of mothers, and children's clinics. The health post was to be staffed by a variety of workers, including a health assistant (who was in charge), sometimes an assistant health worker, and assistant nurse-midwives (ANMs). The ANMs were to provide family planning and maternal and child health services at the post, during outreach clinics, and during regular home visits in the local area. They were also to encourage traditional midwives to participate in these activities. This was the first time in Nepal that assistant nurse-midwives were attached to rural health posts and outreach clinics or expected to make home visits on a regular basis (Nepal/Berkeley 1975:237).

Health inspectors managed the district health office and supervised health post operations by making periodic visits to guide and supervise the staff. The inspectors were never medical doctors, however, and they usually had no clinical training. They could not, therefore, provide the essential technical support to health post staff. Most of them had transferred from the supervisory staff of the malaria project or one of the other vertical projects. The district medical officer, who was the senior doctor in charge of the district hospital, also was expected to supervise the health post staff.

In 1975 an evaluation of the pilot projects, designed and financed mainly by the donor agencies, was carried out by a team recruited from the Nepal government, WHO, and USAID. Both Nepali and foreign advisors indicated in 1979 that there had been considerable controversy about the evaluation; they implied that some of the evaluators were influenced by their desire to continue the integrated program. At the local level, the report also touched on sensitive political issues—whether to terminate the existing vertical programs, each with its own organization and staff, and the international agencies' commitment to promoting the concept of integrated basic health services.

Essentially the evaluation, which focused on technical and service issues, determined that the pilot projects were having serious problems. The USAID contracting team, Health Associates, summarized its conclusions as follows:

> The pilot integrated health posts offered more family planning/maternal and child health services and showed a more efficient expenditure of funds than the nonintegrated health posts. Also, a majority of the families in the pilot districts were visited monthly or bimonthly. On the negative side, even in the pilot project, only five rupees per person was available for health care (one-third for direct service), which is only slightly above the national average. This small amount was seen as a major limiting factor, as improved efficiency could have little effect on such a small amount.
>
> Second, malaria and tuberculosis surveillance and demographic data gathering were poorly done. This was attributed in part to a breakdown in the logistic and information systems and partly to an over-loading of the minimally trained multipurpose worker. The most devastating problem was described as widespread difficulties in personnel, supervision, finance and budget, logistics, and information systems, so that the program was barely functioning only two years after its inception. (Health Associates 1978:15)

Despite the evidence that integration would be difficult to implement, by mid-1975 four more Terai districts (Parsa, Rautahat, Saptari, and Siraha) had started integrated programs on the Bara model, and Kaski District was converted to the Bara model as well. It is not clear from the evaluation report why the more ambitious Bara model was chosen rather than the Kaski model. The Bara model meant the creation of a new infrastructure, with a new category of workers and necessary training programs. The new Division of Integrated Basic Health Services in the Department of Health Services took over the program, setting aside the existing structure of the vertical projects. Because of different educational requirements, most workers from the vertical programs could not be transferred to the Department of Health

Services. New manpower and training problems were therefore created, and the more gradual strategy of incrementally increasing fieldworkers' skills was abandoned.

Thus, one of the original reasons for creating the integrated program—the absorption of malaria workers—was lost. Instead, single-purpose workers were withdrawn from districts that became integrated. Some malaria workers transferred to the integrated program, mainly at the supervisory level, but usually at a lower salary than they had earned before. Basically, the vertical projects were continued, even the Smallpox Eradication Project, which since the eradication of smallpox had been converted into a new vertical project— the Expanded Program of Immunization—with the support of WHO and UNICEF. The malaria project continued as a separate entity because the incidence of malaria was rising again and the newly integrated districts were having difficulty meeting the challenge, especially in the Terai.

Other adjustments were made as the bureaucracy in Kathmandu pressed forward with plans to expand integrated basic health services rapidly. It quickly became clear that expansion would be slowed by limited resources, especially the lack of adequately trained workers. Accordingly, the original plan to integrate fully one district at a time was abandoned in 1975. Instead, phased integration was introduced in several districts simultaneously in an attempt to carry out the government policy of providing expanded services more rapidly to more people—even though this decision further exacerbated the shortage of trained personnel and resources. This strategy yielded distinctions between various stages of integration, from the nonintegrated health post, to the partially integrated post (which had at least some village health workers attached and provided more comprehensive services), to the fully integrated post (which had a full complement of health workers as well as more comprehensive services).

As the integration policy took hold, "integration" took on different meanings in different bureaucratic contexts. For USAID it meant combining the health, population, and nutrition divisions within the USAID organization. For the Nepal government it meant combining vertical programs under a single administration. For some donors it meant combining health services with services in other areas, such as agriculture and education. My interviews with senior members of the Health Ministry revealed that because the meaning of integration was not clear, donors and planners were not always working toward the same goals.

Several Nepalis described their feeling that the international agencies had applied pressure on the Nepali bureaucracy to accept integration. One official said that integration had been the object of an "international hard sell" by WHO and other agencies. A Nepali doctor observed that priorities in health are set by the foreign aid available, and the country follows suit. A member of the Planning Commission described the role of the agencies as imposing a plan on Nepal which had been developed elsewhere; integration did not grow from below, he said, but was imposed from above. Another high-level official said that his predecessor had accepted the integrated approach because the agency involved rewarded him with a job overseas. Many Nepalis gave examples of how they felt they were encouraged to cooperate with agency policies by being given jobs in the agencies or by being invited to attend international meetings.

Not surprisingly, integration met resistance from the system it was designed to replace. The vertical programs strongly resisted it, particularly the malaria and family planning/maternal and child health programs, which were powerful enough to retain their old status. Not only the Nepali staff but also donor agencies assisting the malaria and family planning programs used both financial and informal pressure to support their continuation (American Public Health Association 1980:21). The government, although it officially supported integration, did not provide strong political and administrative leadership for it. Most senior staff assigned to the integrated program were merely on loan from other programs, and thus there was a sense of only temporary administration. Likewise, the small, makeshift office the program occupied, when compared to the larger, better-constructed, better-equipped offices of the vertical programs, seemed to symbolize the government's tentative commitment.

Yet in 1978–79, though it was just a few years old, integration had already become entrenched in its way. One foreign advisor commented that although integration was not working as planned, his agency was committed to assisting it because it represented Nepal government policy. A Nepali official said that even though the Ministry of Health recognized serious problems with integration, it was "boxed in" by foreign aid agreements and had to continue this approach. Whatever the reality of the political, administrative, and implementation problems it presented, integrated basic health services had become Nepal's dominant rural health strategy for the 1970s, and the prime focus of donor assistance.

Integrated Community Health Program and Primary Health Care

As the health bureaucracy in Kathmandu struggled to achieve integration, new ideas were circulating in international health policy circles. In addition to their disappointment with the technological approach to medical care, policymakers now reflected on the disadvantages of health programs that were essentially installed by outside initiative and supported by outside resources. The consensus was that long-term improvement in the health of Third World populations must ultimately depend on greater community participation and self-reliance in health care. In response to the new emphasis on community participation, Nepal's rural health program was given a new name. Integrated Basic Health Services was now called the Integrated Community Health Program (ICHP).[2]

By the late 1970s, community participation had blossomed into a major new concept in international health called primary health care (PHC). WHO and UNICEF, its principal architects, promoted PHC at the highest policy level during the International Conference on PHC at Alma Ata, in the Soviet Union, in 1978.

Primary health care evolved as a concept from the social experiments being carried out in China, North Vietnam, and

Cuba, especially the Chinese model of the "barefoot doctor." The barefoot doctor epitomized the PHC planners' concern for local-level involvement in health care and the use of simple, "appropriate" medical technology.

The "Declaration of Alma Ata" defined primary health care as

> essential health care based on practical, scientifically sound and socially acceptable methods and technology made universally accessible to individuals and families in the community through their full participation and at a cost that the community and country can afford to maintain at every stage of their development in the spirit of self-reliance and self-determination. It forms an integral part of the country's health system, of which it is the central function and main focus, and of the overall social and economic development of community. It is the first level of contact of individuals, the family, and community with the national health system, bringing health care as close as possible to where people live and work, and constitutes the first element of a continuing health care process. (World Health Organization 1978:3–4)

Thus, primary health care is a process that involves all levels of care—a chain of support according to needs based on the following eight essential elements:

1. education concerning prevailing health problems and the methods of preventing and controlling them;

2. promotion of food supply and proper nutrition;

3. an adequate supply of safe water and basic sanitation;

4. maternal and child health care, including family planning;

5. immunization against the major infectious diseases;

6. prevention and control of locally endemic diseases;

7. appropriate treatment of common diseases and injuries;

8. provision of essential drugs. (World Health Organization 1984:5)

Primary health care programs are generally oriented to rural areas; they are designed to require few outside resources. The community receiving services is expected to play an active role in providing, maintaining, and financing them. Since the services must be appropriate to people's specific needs and to the social and economic environment, the precise form of a primary health care system is expected to vary according to local political, economic, social, and cultural patterns. Primary health care differs from basic health care in the locus of responsibility. With basic health care, basic services were provided for communities. With primary health care, the emphasis is on community participation, and communities are expected to be more involved in providing their own services.

By the late 1970s, the PHC approach had been put into effect on a nationwide scale in only a few countries with socialist governments. But since then the international health agencies have been promoting PHC as the solution to the health problems of developed as well as developing countries. The rhetoric and jargon of primary health care are prominent in many recent articles and books on rural health in the Third World, as well as in policy statements and other documents from the international agencies.

In Nepal the donor agencies quickly focused on the primary health care approach. By the time of this research (1978–79), the Integrated Community Health Program was being referred to as primary health care, even though its only substantive difference from the former Integrated Basic Health Services was the addition of the community health volunteer. Donor funds that formerly had been targeted to support integration were now designated for primary health care, but the program they supported was largely the same. Thus, the rural health program's identity was manipulated to fit the latest shift in policy orientation emanating from the international level.

The history of international health aid and its outcomes in Nepal illuminates several important points about the policy-making process:

First, the donor agencies did not adequately investigate the practical implications of new approaches, and they spent too little time in creating the infrastructure for their successful application before promoting them. Primary health care may be theoretically sound, but its practical applicability in Nepal has not yet been demonstrated in other than small-scale projects. "Although the concept of primary health care has strong political support, a strategy for its large-scale implementation has not been devised" (Galladay 1980:ii). Similarly, the agencies pressed ahead with integration on a national scale in Nepal, even though the results of the two-year pilot projects revealed serious problems in implementation.

Second, new policies conceived at the international level are often promoted without sufficient regard to the particular setting in which they are being introduced. In the negotiations between donor agencies and national ministries of health, the outcome is weighted toward the donors because of their overwhelming resources. Thus, Third World recipient countries like Nepal, with their different needs, resources, and cultures, often accept programs that reflect the donor's priorities more than their own. In theory, recipient governments can ask for assistance to meet their national priorities, but national plans are more often adapted to the policies the donors are currently promoting, because funds for programs that fit these policies are readily available. Sometimes international priorities fit the recipient country's circumstances, as in the case of the malaria program, but at other times they do not.

Third, policy changes came too fast and frequently for the Nepali system to absorb them. Within a decade, international policy shifted from vertical approaches, to integrated basic health services, to community participation, to primary health care. By mid-June 1979, the focus of international policy was already shifting away from primary health care toward infant diarrheal-disease control—in effect, a new vertical program. Conferences and reports on infant survival were then receiving priority attention. High-level officials frequently return from international meetings with new policy directives that entail new programs. As the donor agencies move from one approach to the next, recipient countries may be left without support for the discarded structures, programs, and specially trained staff of the old approach. One Nepali planner commented that he thought integration was feasible but that it could not be started "overnight." He felt that it should have been introduced more gradually, taking into account the needs and resources in each district and the technical support that the vertical programs could offer. Fourth, policymakers failed to recognize sufficiently the fragility of systems and the scarcity of resources in Nepal. Thus, a Nepali physician in the Ministry of Health described integration as a logical idea that deserved support, but he questioned how Nepal could be expected to achieve it when there were so few existing rural services to integrate.

The Planning Process

Planning, the essential link between policy and programs, has become a major preoccupation of the international agencies, partly in response to criticisms that early programs were poorly planned. Many hours are spent in the health bureaucracies talking about how to plan, who is to plan, and what is needed to plan. International consultants help governments set up planning agencies, carry out planning workshops, and develop planning kits. At the policymaking stage, which is centered primarily in Geneva and Washington, the international agencies have minimal contact with the Nepal government, but at the planning stage, which for Nepal is centered in Kathmandu, contact is much more frequent. Planning is the setting for extensive interaction between the agencies and the government—interaction that reflects the cultural differences between the bureaucracies. Because planners have little information about rural conditions, health plans tend to reflect priorities in Geneva, Washington, or Kathmandu rather than rural needs and resources.[3]

Country Health Programming

Comprehensive health planning was introduced to Nepal through the country health programming exercise promoted by WHO in 1974. Country health programming was developed at WHO headquarters in Geneva and promoted in Bangladesh and Thailand as well as in Nepal by the WHO Southeast Asia Regional Office. Its purpose was to prepare recipient countries for expanding health services by introducing planning techniques based on concepts of scientific management developed by economists and organizational specialists in business schools. Equally important, it would provide a basis for accountability by identifying the country's priorities in health and setting measurable goals to be achieved. Donors could then judge the effectiveness of their expenditures by measuring the impact of aid on the national health status.

The approach was systematic and comprehensive, embracing an entire country's health needs: as described by WHO, country health programming was "designed to identify priority health problems of prime concern to countries in the context of their development plan; to specify targets in these problem areas; to translate targets into health programmes to be accomplished during a plan period through the identification of activities, resource needs and the organization required to obtain these objectives; and to implement, evaluate and reformulate such programmes on a continuing basis." Another very important objective was to identify where and when foreign assistance would be needed to meet national goals. Social and economic information was to be taken into account: "Throughout the entire process, a strong emphasis was to be placed on the interaction between the health sector and other sectors in the socio-economic field" (WHO 1974:1).

To WHO officials in 1974, the country health programming approach appeared ideally suited to Nepal. Despite the increasing attention paid to the country's health needs during the preceding decade, Nepal had no formal planning agency and no comprehensive health plan. The country health programming exercise could give Nepali planners more experience in international health planning methods, establish health guidelines for the government's fifth five-year development plan (1975–80), and provide a framework for the rapidly increasing donor assistance.

The exercise was conducted in 1974, mainly by planners and systems analysts from WHO headquarters in Geneva and from the Southeast Asia regional office in New Delhi. A number of Nepalis worked with them. A national committee appointed by the Nepal government to carry out country health programming was composed of fifteen members: ten Nepali medical doctors and administrators and five WHO staff members. After the committee's plenary meetings, a smaller committee of five Nepali doctors and six WHO advisors carried out the detailed work. The nine Nepali doctors heading the vertical health projects also assisted, along with at least seven other advisors and consultants from WHO. Since the Nepali participants were all medical doctors and administrators, however, with no experience in comprehensive, multisectoral planning, the numerous WHO experts and consultants contributed all the health planning expertise. The meetings were conducted in English to accommodate the many foreign advisors and consultants participating.

After almost two years of work, the committee presented a two-volume report that described how the exercises had been carried out, charted a course for Nepal's health sector during its fifth five-year development plan, and proposed detailed programs for carrying out this strategy. The report illustrates the international planners' orientation toward quantifiable ("hard") data and targets as opposed to more qualitative social and cultural observations.

Country health programming opened with a workshop for Nepalis conducted by WHO technical staff members, who talked about rationale and methods and prepared a plan for the exercise. The planning itself was carried out in stages. The first stage was devoted to collecting and analyzing quantifiable information. Because little centralized statistical and descriptive data existed, the committee collected new data from various sources, both official and nonofficial. The results could scarcely be considered satisfactory. Since Nepal had no nationwide system for recording cases of illness or for registering births and deaths, morbidity and mortality rates could be only roughly estimated. Also, the data were sharply skewed toward the urban minority, because the urban-based hospitals were the main data source; for lack of records, rural Nepal remained largely unrepresented. Data analysis faced serious obstacles in Kathmandu, where data-processing facilities were limited. For the sake of efficiency, some of the data were sent to WHO headquarters in Geneva for analysis. But this procedure was expensive, and more important, it defeated country health programming's purpose of training Nepali planners in procedures that they could repeat in the future by themselves.

The next stage identified Nepal's high-priority health problems. The country health programming report contains the preliminary and revised lists of health concerns that were considered. A comparison of these lists reveals that during successive editing, the committee eliminated without explanation socially related problems such as inadequate health information and lack of adequate health services. Only an outline of diseases and population growth was retained. According to one WHO advisor, the agency was looking for problems that could be analyzed into specific, quantifiable variables for the purpose of measuring change.

The next stage set targets—quantifiable measures that could be used to show changes in health patterns and health coverage—and devised strategies to meet these targets. Meeting targets was to become the key criterion for the success of rural health programs, despite the difficulty of collecting accurate data in rural Nepal.

In the final stage, the committee prepared plans for programs in the high-priority areas. One of these was Integrated Basic Health Services (later to become the Integrated Community Health Program), which received attention along with Nepal's other high-priority programs—family planning, nutrition, health education, malaria eradication/control, tuberculosis control, leprosy control, smallpox eradication, goiter, water supply, and sanitation–excreta disposal. The plans for each program were extensive and specific, including a detailed program description, manpower requirements, financial implications, and legal provisions. Significantly, Integrated Basic Health Services was treated no differently than the vertical programs in the planning process, even though it was supposed to be gradually incorporating them.[4] Although international policy favoring integration had been acknowledged by the creation of Integrated Basic Health Services, at the national planning level the efforts toward integration were being compromised amid the continuing pressures from interest groups that favored the existing vertical programs.

By 1978–79, the detailed plans produced by the country health programming exercise had been largely abandoned. What had happened to the product of so much thought and effort? Foreign advisors and Nepali health officials alike told me that the plans were unrealistic and could serve only as idealized guidelines. The outcome is not surprising in view of the scanty data on which the plans were based. Several Nepali health officers commented to me that the foreign experts who conducted the country health programming exercise had only a superficial knowledge of Nepal's resources and conditions. Certainly, the foreign experts had little experience in the rural areas that Integrated Basic Health Services was expected to serve. Many of the Nepali participants in country health planning themselves had a limited understanding of rural needs because they were from urban families. Furthermore, the planning process did not allow time to acquire such information. Despite WHO's stated objective of taking social and economic factors into account, no means for accomplishing this had been found.

The planning process demonstrated in the country health programming exercise was itself too sophisticated for the Nepali planners to use as a model in the future—not for lack of imagination and understanding but for lack of information, time, and resources (such as support personnel, office equipment, and data-processing equipment). Nepali participants in the exercise told me that it had been more useful in showing them how to plan according to international formats than in producing usable plans. Some Nepali health officers saw its value as chiefly political. They considered the preparation of sophisticated plans a useful device to obtain foreign assistance—not, as WHO officials intended, an educational device to demonstrate how to assess national health needs and design strategies for meeting them.

Health officials in Kathmandu may have felt detached from the exercise and uncommitted to the resulting programs, since initiative, manpower, and financing were mostly external. Some Nepalis described country health programming to me as a WHO exercise, dominated by foreign experts who had only a superficial knowledge of Nepal's resources and conditions. Certainly it was more compatible with WHO's priorities, resources, and operating procedures than with those of the Nepali health system, and it served WHO's organizational need for detailed plans to justify expenditures more effectively than it served the need for delivering health services in rural Nepal. It did achieve at least one of WHO's objectives, though—to start the health planning process in Nepal.

An assessment of country health programming in Nepal and other countries made by an independent contracting team for USAID came to similar conclusions:

1. Although country health programming teaches participants techniques for designing programs and establishing priorities, it focuses too narrowly on the planning process.

2. As a planning process, it may be too complex and demanding for the limited resources of the least-developed countries.

3. It is often undertaken by a recipient country to draw technical assistance from WHO and to attract increased support from the international donor community, without any desire by the country's ministry of health for comprehensive planning. Health planning activities are often oriented toward donors' priorities and interests, especially their desire to make sure that the increasing amounts of aid they are providing to countries such as Nepal are being effectively spent.

4. Exercises such as country health programming are oriented more toward analyzing and solving problems in the supply of services (that is, facilities and manpower) than toward considering the demand for these services by the population (Family Health Care 1979:45).

Further Planning Efforts

WHO followed the country health programming exercise with the concept of project formulation, which involved further detailed planning for specific projects. This time the objective was both training in planning and the production of workable plans. Accordingly, in 1975 the Nepal government appointed several task forces to prepare detailed programs for the vertical projects and for the Integrated Basic Health Services. More Nepali nationals were involved in this stage, but WHO representatives were on each task force, and one member from WHO's Southeast Asia regional office in New Delhi worked with all of them.

Participating in these task forces was the first experience for the Ministry of Health in detailed operational planning for Integrated Basic Health Services. The task forces worked for three months to develop the operations plan, which covered every aspect from the selection of health post sites (there were to be 810 health posts, equitably distributed throughout the country, by 1980) to staff recruitment, training, and supervision; logistics; supply; information systems; technical inputs; management and health output evaluations; budget considerations; relationships with traditional healers; and inter- and intraministry relationships. The broad concepts developed were "phased integration of vertical project activities (family planning/maternal and child health, malaria, tuberculosis/leprosy, smallpox) and some vertical project staff (both at field and district supervisory levels), emphasizing high-payoff interventions for high-risk groups on a predominantly outreach basis, and with community support." In accordance with the then-current policy in international agencies, planning and implementation were to be somewhat decentralized to the region and district (USAID 1976:17).

Preparing the project formulations for Integrated Basic Health Services was difficult and time-consuming, since essentially it required designing a new system to incorporate five separate vertical projects—those for malaria, family planning/maternal and child health, smallpox, leprosy, and tuberculosis—into basic health services. In retrospect, the plan has been criticized both for being too detailed and for not dealing with the central question of how integration should be achieved, a matter that never has been addressed. A former WHO advisor for Nepal's project formulations said that he was satisfied with the exercise because it set a precedent for detailed planning which he hoped would be followed in the preparation of Nepal's sixth five-year development plan. Nepali officials said, as they also said of country health programming, that the exercise was useful. But in fact, the government never signed the final documents. (The project formulations did have their unofficial uses, though, in answering questions about health programs. When I asked about the structure of various projects, I was usually referred to the project formulations, despite the fact that they were not official.) Finally, neither Nepalis nor foreign advisors considered the project formulations realistic in terms of implementation.

The influence of the international agencies carried over to planning at the national level even when foreign advisors were absent. In 1976, after several long-term health plans had been drafted for the Ministry of Health, a final and official long-term plan was produced by a special committee of the Janch Bhuj Kendra of the Palace Secretariat and presented to the king. Serving on this committee were the chief of the Health Planning Unit (established by the Ministry of Health in 1974), who was a medical doctor, along with another medical doctor and a member of the Ministry of Finance. They worked in isolation from foreign advisors, but the influence of the agencies was reflected in the fact that the committee did not consider any approaches other than integration. The single nonmedical member of the committee told me that he was the only one who encouraged taking social factors into consideration and that the others were oriented to a narrower medical approach.

A more recent example of donor-initiated activity in health planning is the *Country Health Profile on Nepal*, proposed and prepared by WHO in 1978. Prepared mostly by

a WHO advisor with advice from the former Nepali director
of health planning, the profile was published in English and
distributed very selectively to donor agencies and government officials, but not at the district level. It included general
background information on Nepal, a description of the
health administration, national health policies, plans, and
legislation; an assessment of the health situation, resources,
and their utilization; a description of Nepal's participation
in WHO panels and committees; and a list of external
sources of support (WHO 1979). The profile was primarily
desired by foreign planners, who saw this compendium as
the first step in establishing a bank of baseline data on which
change could be measured. The WHO representative, who
had assisted in the production of a similar document in another country, stated that preparing the profile on Nepal had
given him personal satisfaction. But it was decribed by Nepalis as "being for the foreigners," and in fact its value lay in
providing a handy compendium comparing health statuses
throughout the world.

In 1974, shortly after the country health programming exercise had begun, the Nepal government had organized its
own health planning bureaucracy. Responding to a request
by the Planning Commission that planning sections be created in all government ministries to gather data and provide
technical advice, the Ministry of Health established the
Health Planning Unit. The staff of this unit worked on the
later stages of country health programming, the health sector
of the fifth five-year development plan, and the long-term
health plan. USAID and WHO influenced the Health Planning Unit mainly by providing training grants for members
of the Ministry of Health—especially for earning a master's
degree in public health in the United States—and by assigning foreign advisors to the unit.

During the time of this research (1978–79), the Health
Planning Unit consisted of a planning chief, an assistant
chief, three section officers, and two expatriate advisors.
Only the assistant chief had formal training in health plan-
ning, obtained from a short course at the Johns Hopkins
School of Public Health in Baltimore. Since general policy

and plans were formulated by the National Planning Commission, the planning unit's work was largely routine, including such tasks as preparing annual plans and making quarterly evaluations of Ministry of Health projects. The planning unit also prepared some technical reports at the request of the National Planning Commission.

In 1978–79, the planning unit was much involved in preparing the annual plan and in organizing and participating in the task forces for Nepal's sixth five-year development plan. It was also coordinating the Midterm Review of the health activities of the fifth five-year plan. The Nepal government, WHO, the United Nations Fund for Population Activities (UNFPA), UNICEF, and USAID financed and conducted this evaluation, the first such attempt in Nepal. Planners hoped that it would indicate how the health sector's performance could be improved and would provide a more comprehensive and quantitative data base for future planning and management decisions (Nepal Ministry of Health 1979:11). The areas covered represented the full range of the health sector's organization and activities, including its resources, its organizational processes, the services provided, and the response from the Nepali population.

The midterm review, which was under way while I was in Nepal, was an ambitious and important undertaking because it was the first systematic attempt to send workers to rural areas to survey health services and conditions. The difficulties the project encountered illustrate the administrative and practical obstacles to gathering data in Nepal. First, despite the active participation of AID consultants, none of the advisors who worked on the midterm review were experienced in conducting survey research. They did not know how to construct questionnaires for use in the field. Second, language differences were a continuing problem. Questionnaires prepared in English had to be translated into Nepali and subsequently into other languages spoken in various local areas to be surveyed. Workers who spoke the local language had to be found and trained for each area. Third, delays in funding approval by the government and the agencies set the survey schedule back into the monsoon season. Fieldwork was extremely difficult to carry out with the roads and footpaths blocked, the rivers swollen, and the airports closed.

Several Nepali health officials were involved in the early stages of the midterm health review, but later more and more of the actual work was done by the advisors from USAID and WHO. The review was referred to by other foreigners and by Nepalis as an evaluation by USAID, since the USAID advisors were the most visible actors as designers and analyzers of the data, and AID was one of the principal financers. The advisors were sensitive about this label because it identified the program with their foreign group rather than more appropriately with the Nepal government. Again, the data were taken out of the country for computer analysis, a time-consuming measure and an inappropriate one if the agencies wanted to establish evaluation methods that could be repeated in Nepal in the future.

Work on the project formulations, the long-term health plan, and the fifth five-year health plan was proceeding simultaneously in 1975. Planners had intended that each of these exercises would build on information from its predecessors. Because all procedures were taking place at the same time, however, an orderly progression was not possible. Some information and experiences were communicated by informal links, since many of the same people had worked on all three projects. Similar cross-fertilization took place in 1979, when the midterm review and planning for the sixth five-year development plan were in progress.

Planning exercises in Nepal have typically produced planning documents that may not be considered useful by government officers but that satisfy the sponsoring agency's needs. All too often the contents of the plans have been either too complex for the Nepali infrastructure to carry out or simply unrealistic in view of local conditions. The case of the community health volunteer program illustrates how information gaps and failures of cultural understanding prevent policymakers and planners from dealing effectively with conditions in rural villages.

Planning for Community Participation: A Case Example

According to the international health policy of the late 1970s, community participation was necessary to make rural health programs work. In defining primary health care, Dr. Halfdan Mahler, Director-General of the World Health Organization, stated that "such a system will be a kind that countries can afford, provided that villagers and townsfolk themselves participate actively in it, and contribute to it in labor and in kind" (Mahler 1978:3). Thus, community participation was a basic concept in primary health care planning, the major focus of WHO, USAID, and UNICEF in 1978–79; in Nepal it was expected to transform the Integrated Community Health Program into primary health care.

The international agencies promoted the concept of community participation at the regional WHO/UNICEF primary health care conferences, held in both Nepal and New Delhi in 1977, and also at the international Alma Ata conference in 1978, to which a team of Nepalis was invited. The agencies also promoted the concept by funding regional and local workshops, offering training grants, providing technical health consultants and advisors, and giving direct financial assistance.

In one approach to community participation, the community was to choose one of its members who, after a short training course, would attend to its priority health needs. This idea, strongly promoted by WHO, was adopted by health planners in Nepal. There it was translated into a program for the selection and training of unpaid community-level health volunteers who would spread information about health programs and assist the paid village health workers.

As a consequence of the Alma Ata conference, international interest in health volunteers escalated in the late 1970s. Numerous advisors and extensive financial assistance became available for health volunteers in Nepal by the spring of 1979. In addition to the many international agencies and foundations that were already assisting the primary health care program, many others were negotiating with the government and competing for an opportunity to fund aspects of training programs for community health volunteers. There appeared to be not only a lack of coordination but also some competition among donors. The United Nations and bilateral and private donors were all ready to fund and advise on the same aspects of the program, often without considering how their efforts fit in with the present government efforts and with those of other donors. To make matters even more confusing, some donors were working directly with the Department of Health Services, and others were working through Nepali voluntary agencies represented by the Nepal Red Cross, which was interested in training community volunteers but had limited experience in doing so. USAID, which funded advisors to ICHP on training and community participation, was at the same time assisting and financing a private voluntary group from the United States that wanted to start training institutions for village volunteers in the far western area of Nepal.

The agencies' bandwagon approach was further reflected in the policy guidelines given to the Ministry of Health by the National Planning Commission for Nepal's sixth five-year plan (1980–85). These guidelines gave continued support to expanding integrated health services in rural areas, and they also added two new objectives: (1) decentralizing the planning and implementation of health projects to the district level, and (2) training and placing 30,000 community health volunteers within the sixth five-year plan. During task force meetings on health recommendations for the sixth plan, much of the discussion focused on how to define the tasks of community health volunteers, how to recruit and train them, and how to initiate and implement a program with 30,000 volunteers over the next five years, since at that time no program existed. Ambitious programs such as this— strongly promoted and influenced by donors and frequently adopted for local political reasons—have contributed to unrealistic plans and targets, with resulting problems in implementation.

The first actual planning for community participation in health began in Nepal when UNFPA budgeted some funds for training community leaders as part of its assistance to integrated health. Since there was no community participation program yet, the funds were not spent, but they were carried forward and rebudgeted for the next three years. Then, following WHO/UNICEF-sponsored conferences in both Nepal and Delhi in 1977, in which community participation was promoted, the Nepali doctor from ICHP who had attended these meetings instructed one of the training officers to start a community volunteer program. The officer was given no guidance other than that he should prepare a budget for funding 2,000 to 3,000 community volunteers in forty-eight of the seventy-five districts, the number being determined by the money budgeted through UNFPA, not by what was possible.

A foreign advisor attached to ICHP saw his Nepali colleague working on this budget and inquired about it. According to the advisor, he then tried to work with the ICHP training staff to find out what the volunteers would be expected to do and what they would need in order to do it. This group developed a preliminary proposal and planned to conduct two pilot studies for selecting and training health volunteers. Two pilot areas were chosen in the Terai and in the hills, but because the king was planning to make a regional visit to the far western area of Nepal, a third pilot area was added in the west. Training materials were quickly developed and volunteers were recruited, all within a few months. Since that time, attempts have been made to revise these materials and to review implementation problems, which include such basic issues as budgeting, selecting personnel, and preparing job descriptions.

Although the central training officers tried to conduct follow-up and evaluation in the pilot districts, it was difficult for them to get feedback because all three pilot districts had personnel problems similar to those underlying ICHP in general. In one district, no health inspector was assigned, and so there was no one to conduct the training sessions; in another district, a health inspector was posted months late; and in the third, the health inspector would not conduct the volunteer training without receiving advance allowances for daily expenses and travel.

Despite these problems, in August 1978 all health inspectors were called to Kathmandu for a three-day workshop on training volunteers. Unfortunately, the workshop was called hastily and without enough preparation to make training effective; the training materials were not even ready in time. In this respect, the workshop was described by one organizer as a disaster, although the training officers did learn something about what was needed locally from discussions with the health inspectors.

The training officers and the consultant concluded that the panchayat and ward representatives were interested in having the program and were only waiting for guidance. They followed through by distributing money, materials, and instructions to health inspectors for conducting training sessions at fifty-nine health posts in twenty-three districts. Training sessions were carried out in many areas, although the Ministry of Health had not yet decided on a final job description for the health volunteers or on whether they would be paid. Again, there was very little follow-up about health workers' experiences in the field or about how the participants in the training program responded to it.

Although the advisors involved in the pilot phase of the program advised the training officers to proceed slowly, the Nepalis in ICHP were under pressure from the government and other international advisors to produce results rapidly. The community participation concept had spread quickly because it was supported by a wide range of groups. It was a high priority of most international health agencies and of the Nepal government. In addition to the strong promotional and financial influence from the donor agencies, ICHP was under pressure from the Palace and from the prestigious Social Service Coordination Committee (which was under the leadership of a member of the Royal Family) to develop community involvement in the form of community health volunteers. A third source of pressure was the Planning Commission's policy statement that there should be a community health volunteer in every village, or 30,000 volunteers, by 1985. As a result of these multiple pressures, the community participation concept was seized upon, developed, and expanded without any real proof that it was viable.

The need for training materials presented another circumstance in which the availability of funds seemed to be the impetus for hasty action. In 1979, ICHP decided to use WHO money to develop a manual for use by health volunteers. The manual, developed very quickly, was a translation of *Where There Is No Doctor*, itself a translation of *Donde No Hay Doctor*, a manual developed in Mexico by David Werner (1977) for use outside government health services. Although Nepali diagrams were substituted for those in the original text, little time was given to considering whether the manual was appropriate for Nepal or would serve its intended purpose. Its introduction implicitly required the community health volunteer to be able to read easily. My research assistant attended two health post sessions where this manual was used by district health inspectors to train potential volunteers. He observed that even the village elite, most of whom had some education, had considerable difficulty in reading and understanding it.

The remaining money allocated by WHO for community participation activities was spent for a conference held in March 1979 to discuss the training of community health volunteers. Kathmandu officials place great importance on high-level conferences because they are a visible activity that extends legitimacy to programs such as ICHP. This conference was very timely politically, since it coincided with several other meetings taking place on the sixth five-year development plan, in which opposition to integration was expected from employees of vertical health projects.

The conference, proposed as a working seminar, was typical of others sponsored by the Department of Health Services. Although some health inspectors and health workers from the districts were invited to participate, the proceedings were dominated by a number of very senior officials who gave speeches and attended for short periods of time. The Minister of Health opened the conference. Others who gave major addresses were members of the National Planning Commission and the National Panchayat *(Rastriya Panchayat)*, along with several senior doctors from Tribhuvan University and from the health establishment in Kathmandu.

The participation of elites gave legitimacy to the seminar and strengthened its political effectiveness, but it also intimidated less senior participants from the rural areas, who could speak only to local conditions. Since the senior men were too busy to review training materials and did not have time to remain for discussion, the sessions had little continuity. Health inspectors who did speak out told me afterward that they did not think the senior officials had been interested in what they had had to say or would take action on the points they had raised. They felt that they had been invited to be told what to do rather than to supply information based on their experience. The seminar did break up into small discussion groups for part of each day, but again the senior leaders dominated. Much of the discussion reflected a lack of understanding on the part of senior Nepali officials about rural resources and the realities of local health services, and especially about what responsibilities would be appropriate for a community health volunteer.

Although apparently no one in the planning community had investigated past experiences with community participation in Nepal or had considered whether the country had a tradition of volunteerism, the planners in Kathmandu assumed that community participation would work. Unfortunately, experience indicates otherwise, as a look at the local health committees will suggest. The original ICHP program formulation drafted in 1975 by the government and WHO specified that each integrated health post would be supported by a health committee composed of panchayat members, other local leaders, and the health post staff. This committee's purpose was to support health post services and to promote community involvement in health activities. On my visits to health posts I found that many had no committees. Where committees did exist, they usually met as infrequently as once or twice a year, and most villagers did not know about them. The exception was in areas where a new health post was being constructed. There, the health committee was actively involved in obtaining local labor and supplies to supplement those contributed by the government and also in supervising the construction and budget. The general lack of popular support for such committees provides little evidence that villagers were willing to take an active role in government-initiated health programs.

In 1979, the health planning task force—whose members included all the vertical health project chiefs and representatives from the Health Planning Unit and the Planning Commission—focused on expanding the village health worker's role and on developing and training community health volunteers. Judging from the job description developed for the health volunteer, no attention was paid to the disinterest displayed by local health committees. In brief, the volunteer's duties encompassed motivation work (encouraging villagers to make use of the health facilities, have their children vaccinated, take malaria-preventive measures, take prescribed medicines, and use birth control measures); education (in proper nutrition, sanitation, family planning, home delivery techniques, and the use of rehydration fluid to treat diarrhea); diagnosis (of tuberculosis, leprosy, and malnutrition); treatment (of fever cases and of patients requiring first aid); administration (helping to establish the local vaccination clinic, arranging health education classes and exhibits, helping to form the health committee and serving as its secretary, and gathering statistics on births and deaths); and persuading traditional birth attendants to seek training. All of this was supposed to be accomplished in six hours of unpaid time per week! (See Appendix 3: Functions of Community Health Volunteer.)

Beyond the obviously unrealistic time constraints, the volunteer's job description presented a number of problems. First, people in the hills are farmers and are generally poor. Thus, there was considerable question of their being able to afford to take time from agricultural work to volunteer their services in this way. Second, volunteers were expected to assist and be supervised by village health workers, who themselves performed many of these same functions as full-time employees for a salary averaging 200 rupees per month. In addition the supervision of village health workers by health post staff and district health officers was itself inadequate. Third, in order to carry out their duties, volunteers would need to acquire skills beyond the level of village health workers. And finally, health volunteers would have difficulty, as did village health workers, in carrying out duties that required distributing drugs (which were always in short supply) without adequate training in drug distribution.

The community health volunteer program reveals a chain of events extending from policies promoted in international health agencies to the pressures on planners in Kathmandu and ultimately to unrealistic programs installed at the village level. With little reflection on what community participation might mean in Nepal, or examination of the problems it had encountered in the community development and agriculture extension programs of the 1950s and 1960s (Foster 1981), attention and resources were shifted to the new approach.

4

Delivering Services to Rural Villages

Because integration was being phased in during the late 1970s, health posts varied considerably in the range of services provided. Broadly speaking, they can be divided into three categories: nonintegrated, partially integrated, and fully integrated. Nonintegrated posts had not yet assumed any responsibilities from the vertical projects; they simply provided treatment for common illnesses. Partially integrated posts had assumed some vertical project responsibilities and had village health workers attached to them to provide outreach services. Fully integrated posts provided all services, including those formerly covered by the vertical projects. In 1978–79, Nepal had 533 health posts: 185 were nonintegrated, 283 were partially integrated, and 65 were fully integrated. Of Nepal's seventy-five districts, twenty-three had either partially or fully integrated posts (American Public Health Association 1980:29).

Health posts were organized by population and geographical area. In 1978, most served an average of 30,000 people, although ICHP plans called for 7,000 people to be served by each health post in mountainous areas, 13,000 in the hills, and 25,000 in the Terai. The Department of Health Services had further divided its most peripheral service area into *veks*, which averaged one and a half *panchayats.* (The term *panchayat* was applied not only to government councils but also to the primary political unit in Nepal, which averaged from 3,000 to 5,000 people.) Each health post served four to six *veks;* as integration proceeded, each *vek* ideally was assigned a village health worker (VHW), a paid ICHP employee who circulated from house to house gathering data on health status, identifying health problems, and encouraging villagers to seek care at the post.

The VHWs were supervised at the post by the health assistant, a worker who treated patients and also managed all health post operations. The health assistant was supervised in turn by the health inspector from the district office. Nonintegrated posts had a health assistant but no VHWs. Partially integrated posts had at least a health assistant and some VHWs attached. Fully integrated posts had a number of additional staff members with various levels of paramedical training. All posts had at least one peon, the lowest-ranking worker, whose job was to do custodial work and run errands.

To find out how the policies and plans developed at the international and national levels were affecting health care in Nepal's villages, I visited twenty-four health posts in ten districts during 1978–79—some fully integrated, some partially integrated, and some nonintegrated. My visits revealed that some posts were functioning more effectively than others, often owing to the efforts of exceptional health workers. All posts were struggling with a variety of common problems.

A Partially Integrated Health Post

Among the health posts I visited, Tate Health Post in District I (pseudonyms are used where possible, especially for health posts and districts) was one of the best. In 1979, it was in an early stage of integration, meaning that it was staffed by a health assistant and a peon, with three village health workers attached. It was expected to deal with all health-related problems except malaria surveillance, which was still carried out by the Malaria Eradication Program.

Tate Health Post was located on a ridge at a 4,300-foot elevation on a main trail. To reach it I took a three-hour bus ride from Kathmandu, walked four hours along steep trails to District I headquarters, and then walked another four hours to the post. The health post and the local panchayat shared a three-room building, which the panchayat had constructed with mud and stones. A new building was being constructed for the post by the panchayat with voluntary labor.

The Tate Post served about 19,000 people—7,000 people in Tate panchayat and 12,000 in two other panchayats. Most lived by subsistence farming; in the countryside surrounding the post, rice, corn, and wheat grew in terraced fields. The local population consisted of several castes and ethnic groups: Brahman, Chetri, Tamang, Gurung, Newar, and Magar. Each ethnic group spoke a different language, making it difficult for many patients to communicate with health workers. In this hilly area, some patients walked five hours to reach the post. Those who could not walk were carried in back-baskets or on stretchers.

Tate was known as the best health post in the district, mainly because of its active health assistant, a twenty-four-year-old Newar man. He had had a tenth-grade education, followed by two and a half years of training at the Institute of Medicine in Kathmandu, which had included clinical experience in Kathmandu hospitals but no experience at a health post. He was an excellent worker who appeared committed to his work and who had established good rapport with the villagers and local elites. He lived with the family of a local schoolteacher in Tate. Since he was one of the few health assistants who came from a rural hill area, he did not mind Tate's remote location. At the time of my research (in February 1979) he had lived in Tate for five months, but six months later he was transferred to a post located near his family home. Frequent transfers were common practice in the health service.

The Tate health assistant examined, diagnosed, and

treated patients, prescribed medicine, dealt with emergency cases, and worked with the local health committee and panchayat. He also supervised the village health workers, reviewing both their work in the field and their patient registers each month, and prepared all statistics for the district health office. By personality and intelligence, he was well qualified for his work, but because of limited supplies and medicines, and lack of support from district headquarters and Kathmandu, he was unable to accomplish everything his job description and his own standards required. Often, he was unable to give medicine for even common illnesses or to carry out simple suturing of wounds. He told me that he was frustrated by the lack of support for both his routine work and his more innovative ideas.

The other worker who could usually be found at the post was the peon. All government offices have peons, who are at the lowest level in the bureaucracy. At the post the peon's duties were to clean the post and compound area, serve as night watchman, carry messages and supplies between the post and the district headquarters, make tea for the staff, and do anything else his supervisors might ask.

The peon at Tate Health Post was a twenty-four-year-old Magar from the village of Tate. He was the third of five sons and had two younger sisters. Married and the father of a six-month-old son, he had no formal education, although the former health assistant had taught him how to sign his name. Three years earlier, he had heard that a health post would be opened in Tate and had applied successfully for the peon position. Although he described the job as hard work for a low salary (168 rupees monthly, equivalent to about fifteen U.S. dollars), he felt that he had no other choice. Jobs were scarce, especially for an uneducated person, and this job had the advantage of being located near his home. He was busy at the post most of the time. At night he slept there to serve as watchman, even though the post had no mattress or blanket. His only free day was Saturday, when he could stay home and tend his fields.

The peon's day began at about six A.M., when he went for water with the *gagro* (water container), a chore that took about twenty minutes. He transferred some of the water to the filter and cleaned the clinic room and compound. He then joined his family for the morning rice meal and returned to the post at about nine A.M. to open the clinic room, put up the screen, and assemble the equipment. The health post was well arranged, with a desk for the health assistant, a stool for patients, a bench for those waiting, and a small table (where the peon sat) that held the most commonly used medicines and injection equipment. Behind the peon was a shelf with other medicines. When the clinic opened, the peon gave injections, cleaned and dressed wounds, and distributed medicines. Although treating patients was not in his job description, he had learned these skills from the former health assistant. The room arrangement allowed the health assistant to supervise the peon, and the two men appeared to have a very good working relationship. The peon also saw patients who came when the health post was closed, or sent for the health assistant as necessary. When the health assistant was in the field for supervision two days a week, the peon stayed at the post alone, doing simple diagnosis, giving injections, distributing medicines, and taking care of emergencies. At the time of my visit, the health assistant was about to take ten days of official leave. During his absence the peon would be the only worker at the post. In addition to his other duties, the peon frequently carried messages to the village health workers in the field and to district headquarters. While I was at the post, he was sent on a private call to give an injection to an elderly woman, the mother of a panchayat member, who lived about an hour's walk away.

The three village health workers (VHWs) attached to the post were all men, ages twenty-one, twenty-five, and thirty-three. All had eighth-grade educations, and all were from nearby panchayats, located four to eight hours' walk away. They had received four weeks of inservice training in Pathlaiya Training Center which they described as theoretical, not practical. Although they were expected to make sputum smears to detect tuberculosis, for example, they had not been shown how to do this during training but only later at the health post. According to their job description, each

VHW was expected to visit thirty houses daily (painting the date of the visit on the outside of each house), to record vital statistics about family members in a register, and to disseminate health information. If there was any need for care or medication, the VHWs could only refer patients to the health post, since they were not trained to dress wounds, diagnose diseases, or give medicine. In some panchayats, a few simple medicines for worms, aspirin, and vitamins were being given to the VHWs for distribution, but the supply was very limited. (See Appendix 3: Job Description for Village Health Worker.)

Their job was very difficult and had few rewards. In most areas it was physically impossible to visit thirty houses a day and still have time for any motivational work. Houses were often ten to thirty minutes' walk apart, scattered on hillsides and separated by terraced fields. In reality, the VHWs could do little more than paint the date on each house for the benefit of future supervisory visits from the health assistant and record basic data in the register. Villagers often asked why they came, since they could not even give medicine for fever, diarrhea, worms, or headaches.

In Tate patients were usually waiting for the health post to open at ten A.M.; the post closed at three P.M. (official government hours). Between ten and thirty patients came daily, with an average of 250 to 300 monthly, depending on the season. I was there in February, a dry month that is not an especially busy time for farmers. During the planting and harvesting seasons, patients rarely take time to come to the health post, even if they are very ill; during the monsoon season, although the incidence of illness is high, landslides and flooding prevent them from seeking health care.

Most health posts are similar to Tate, staffed by only a health assistant or an assistant health worker and a peon, with some village health workers attached. In the six districts that were fully integrated, health posts had larger staffs—a health assistant, sometimes one or two assistant health workers, an assistant nurse-midwife (ANM), a *mukhiya* (clerk) to do the clerical work, peons, and village health workers for outreach services.

A Fully Integrated Health Post

District II, a former ICHP pilot district, was fully integrated. Of its thirteen health posts, Chittre was the most completely staffed and was reputed to be the best. It was located in Chittre village on a 4,000-foot ridge with a spectacular view of Machha Puchaare and the Annapurna peaks, about three hours' uphill walk from the district headquarters. Chittre was a Brahman and Chetri village, although Chittre panchayat's population was a mixture of castes and ethnic groups, with a majority of Gurungs. The health post occupied the former panchayat building, a four-room stone-and-cement structure, but it was scheduled to move to a newly constructed cement building in a few months. The central government had provided 75 percent of the financing and supplies for the new health post, and the panchayat had contributed 25 percent in local materials and voluntary labor.

Fourteen staff members were assigned to Chittre health post: a health assistant who was the senior member in charge of all activities, two assistant health workers, two assistant nurse-midwives (ANMs), one *mukhiya* (clerk), five village health workers, and three peons. The health assistant, one assistant health worker, and one VHW slept in rooms above the clinic and ate in the village tea stall. The two ANMs slept and cooked their meals in a *dera* (a rented room), ten minutes' walk from the health post, which they rented from a Brahman family. The second assistant health worker and his wife lived in a rented room in a house adjoining the health post. The other staff members lived locally with their families.

On the average, sixty patients came to the post daily, double the usual maximum number in Tate. The area was very hilly, and some patients had to walk seven hours to reach the post. Because of Chittre's proximity to the district headquarters, which is in one of Nepal's largest valleys, many patients bypassed the post, preferring to go to the zonal hospital, a local mission hospital, or to one of the many private clinics and doctors in the district town. The southeastern side of Chittre panchayat is close to an Ayurvedic clinic and to another health post. People in this area usually attended whichever health post was nearest to their home.

Chittre was the first assignment for the health assistant, a twenty-one-year-old Brahman from Kathmandu. He had completed the tenth grade and then had taken two and a half years of training at the Institute of Medicine in Kathmandu. In addition to treating patients, he managed the health post and supervised the staff. He said that his clinical training had been good but that it had not prepared him for his fieldwork responsibilities. He liked examining patients in the clinic but not visiting patients, supervising VHWs in the field, or completing the extensive paperwork required. Although he was scheduled to be in the field ten days a month, he rarely went more than once a month.

After having served for nine months in Chittre, he was eager to be transferred to Kathmandu or to obtain entrance to the new rural doctor program at the Institute of Medicine. He was not optimistic about his chances to succeed in either, since he had no "source or force"—friends or relatives in high government positions who could help him. The same reason was given by the assistant health workers and VHW, among other workers, when speculating about their limited prospects for promotion or transfer to a more desirable area.

The assistant health worker for curative work was stationed primarily at the health post to examine patients. He was twenty-three years old and from Kathmandu, but he had already adjusted to village life. His training included field experience in Palpa District at Tansen Health Worker Training School, which was headed by a foreign mission doctor seconded to the government. Because the Tansen mission hospital staff had worked extensively in remote areas, this school emphasized field experience. The assistant health worker/curative was very competent clinically, had good relationships with patients and villagers, and actually appeared to be more confident and competent than the health assistant. He had had two years' experience in a leprosy hospital before his assignment to Chittre in 1977. When the health assistant examined patients, the assistant health worker/curative gave injections and distributed medicine, but frequently the assistant health worker was left in charge of the clinic and examined patients himself. He went to the field to supervise VHWs about one day a month.

The assistant health worker for preventive health was a forty-five-year-old Newar man from Kathmandu who had worked with the malaria program for seventeen years. Four years earlier, after three weeks of retraining in the integration program, he had been transferred to Chittre Health Post. He had a tenth-grade education and no clinical training. He described his responsibilities as fieldwork, which he felt he did not get credit for because it was harder for supervisors to evaluate than clinical work. Although he said that the extensive walking necessary made his job difficult, others on the staff said that he had very little to do. He frequently applied for transfer to Kathmandu, where his family lived, but he complained that he could not succeed without "source and force." He would have preferred a job in the malaria program, where the salary and benefits were better and the work was more relevant to his experience and training.

Chittre was the only one of the twenty-four posts I visited where two assistant nurse-midwives (ANMs) had been working for an extended period; one had been there for four years, the other for two. Both young women, ages twenty-three and nineteen, were from the district center. Chittre's proximity to their home, which allowed for frequent visits, and the fact that they had found a suitable living arrangement with a family near the post may have contributed to the length of their stay. ANMs often leave their posts early because it is not socially acceptable for young women to live away from home. These two ANMs had completed the eighth grade, followed by a two-year ANM training course. They assisted in the clinic, conducted maternal and child health clinics, and walked together to nearby villages, where they provided ante- and postnatal care and child care and made follow-up visits to clinic patients. They were called upon to assist with two difficult deliveries during my stay in Chittre, but according to the records, they had assisted with only ten home deliveries and one health post delivery during the previous year. Most women delivered at home alone or assisted by a family member. *Dhais* or *sudenis* (traditional midwives) were not found in this region or in many other areas of Nepal.[1]

The *mukhiya* (clerk), twenty-two years old and from Chittre, had worked at the post since it had opened six years earlier. His salary was low (204 rupees monthly), but he kept his job because it was near his home. His responsibilities included administration, handling correspondence with the district and central health offices, sending monthly reports to the district health office, and supervising the clinic storeroom and drug supply. He was supervised by the district accountant, whose most recent visit to the post had been eight months earlier.

The three peons—a woman and two men, all in their twenties—were from Chittre and had worked at the health post for three to five years. They described their main responsibilities as cleaning the health post, collecting malaria blood samples and reports from VHWs in the field, and serving as messengers between Chittre and the district headquarters. The female peon frequently accompanied the ANMs on home visits. Although patient care was not part of their job description, I observed peons cleaning and dressing wounds, and the female peon gave an injection to a patient who came on a holiday when all other staff were away.

The VHWs were from Chittre or nearby panchayats and had backgrounds similar to those of the Tate VHWs. Their additional responsibilities at the fully integrated health post included malaria surveillance and the collection of blood samples.

My observation of the Chittre health post left me with the impression that at most times it was overstaffed for the existing range of activities and supplies. In theory, all staff members had a full work load, but in practice, they spent much of the time sitting in the sun. During the first few days of my visit, the staff members were preoccupied with reports on a series of special mobile immunization clinics that had been held the week before. The VHWs had motivated people to come to the five field clinics, and the assistant health worker for prevention, two ANMs, and peons had conducted them. The statistical reports covered the number of immunizations given and special equipment used. After the reports and unused supplies were sent to the district health office, the post was relatively quiet. The VHWs returned to the field, the mukhiya and assistant health worker for prevention resumed supervising the construction of the new health post, and other staff were frequently away from the clinic or relaxing outside. The clinic's busiest times were at ten A.M., when it opened, and in the early afternoon, when patients who had walked long distances to reach the post arrived. Accidents and emergencies were frequent. When appropriate supplies and medicines were available, patients were treated quickly; but because supplies and medicines often were not available, many patients were referred to the zonal hospital, four hours' walk away.

The Local Panchayat

The Chittre panchayat was the most active one I visited, partly because of the local panchayat member, who was also a member of the district panchayat. He had received awards from the king for outstanding community service and was working to make Chittre a model panchayat. He had initiated several development projects: bringing piped water into the village and constructing a school, a new health post, and a panchayat building. He had proposed a plan for obtaining and distributing drugs. He was a member of the local health committee, which had last met two months earlier to discuss the health post construction.

The Chittre panchayat met on the first day of the Nepali month. The meetings were open to everyone, and I attended. Seventeen men were there, ten of them panchayat members; the one woman panchayat member required by law was not present. The *Pradhan Panch*, president of the Chittre panchayat, chaired the meeting, but the district panchayat was most active in keeping discussion confined to the agenda. After his early departure, the discussion turned to a general unstructured conversation. The agenda included income and expenses of the panchayat; notices and letters from the district and central levels; consideration of a scholarship for a poor high school student; the need for stone for the new school; the sixth five-year development plan; and health post construction. The health post mukhiya explained that a panchayat member must be assigned to supervise the local contribution of stone, since inappropriate stone had been supplied by local residents. Volunteers were needed to transport fifty packets of cement. After much discussion, it was decided that the cement was too heavy for men to carry and would be brought by mule. One of the wards would supply and transport wood for windows and doors. The panchayat had earlier paid 158 rupees to a man in another panchayat to cut the wood, but he had neither done the job nor returned the money. The wards were also required to send volunteer laborers to work on the construction site, although it was not clear how these volunteers would be selected. Often volunteers actually were appointed or ordered by panchayat leaders and local elites to work on development projects. There was no further discussion of problems at the health post. As in other panchayats, the health post committee and panchayat dealt much more readily with health post construction than with other problems in delivering health services. In my discussions with high-level officials in the Ministry of Health, I discovered that few were familiar with how local panchayats actually operated, even though they relied on the panchayat as the locus of community participation.

Shortages

Patients and staff at every health post I visited cited lack of medicine and supplies as the post's main problem. The shortages were especially demoralizing for VHWs, whose primary responsibility was to motivate villagers to come to the post. Patients following this advice often arrived at the post only to be told that there was no medicine. The post and the VHW were thus discredited, and the VHW became the target for the disappointed patients' hostility when he next visited their village. Many clinic staff and local leaders said that until services were reliably available, people should not be encouraged to go to the post. The clinic staff likewise became frustrated, since they could not perform most services without at least simple medicine and equipment. This situation contributed to their dissatisfaction and desire for transfer.

During 1978–79 the government's yearly drug supply ran out after three months because of the limited budget allocated for purchasing costly imported drugs. At all twenty-four of the health posts I visited, drugs were in very short supply. When drugs were available from the government, they were distributed in equal quantities to all health posts. Tate and Chittre thus received the same amount, even though Chittre had twice as many patients.

In Chittre the king had provided drugs as part of a special panchayat flood-relief program in 1976. These extra drugs had been distributed by the health post between 1976 and 1979, building up patients' expectations about their availability. While I was there this special supply was used up. The last anesthetic injection was given during my visit, and thereafter the staff was unable to suture wounds. Some supplies remained from UNICEF's drug supplement of vitamins, worm medicine, aspirin, and gentian violet. Patients were given prescriptions for other drugs and told to purchase them in the district headquarters, since there were no pharmacies in the village. The tea stall stocked a few simple drugs, but they were too expensive for most people in this poor area. The local representative to the district panchayat proposed that Chittre panchayat purchase drugs to be sold through the agriculture cooperative, at cost plus the transport charges, rather than the usual 200 percent retail markup on most drugs sold commercially. If successful, this innovative scheme could be a model for the district.

Since drug shortages were common throughout Nepal, the donor agencies had turned their attention to the problem. UNICEF, in addition to supplying a package of drugs and vitamins for maternal and child health to health posts, was assisting the government with equipment for manufacturing simple drugs in Kathmandu. Representatives of USAID and the Dutch government were also considering giving Nepal assistance for the supply and local manufacture of drugs. Britain Nepal Medical Trust, a small voluntary group initially working on tuberculosis control in eastern Nepal, identified drug shortages in the hill areas as the health system's primary problem (Clugston 1978). To supplement the supply, the Trust developed a scheme for distributing low-cost essential drugs in the hill areas through existing local commercial outlets and local panchayats. It was also working with government officials in eastern districts to improve the distribution of drugs to health posts and hospitals.

The Villagers' Response to Services

In the Chittre area patients did go to the health post for treatment if the post was accessible and if both staff and medicines were available. The most common illnesses were coughs, colds, bronchitis, skin diseases, stomach disorders, jaundice, fever, worms, and goiter. Whatever their symptoms, patients showed a strong preference for injections, believing that they were not being treated properly without them.

For most illnesses patients reported that they "waited in the house to get well." Herbal remedies and dietary regimes were widely used. If illnesses persisted, the next resort was traditional healers—*jhankris, jharnes,* and *fuknes.* Health posts and district hospitals were the last resort, usually sought only for serious and persistent illnesses. Frequently, when the health post was unable to treat a patient successfully, the patient consulted the jhankri again or returned to using herbal medicine.[2]

Nepalis willingly used both traditional and modern medicine. It often appeared that only planners and government health practitioners perceived conflict between different medical systems. Interviews with patients in Chittre and other districts showed that those who did seek treatment at health facilities chose the facility because of location and quality of care rather than type of medical system. If the Ayurvedic clinic was close by, the patient went there rather than to the health post, even though the system and medications differed. Medicines were usually available at Ayurvedic clinics, since they were produced in Nepal and were therefore less expensive than imported allopathic drugs; in addition, Ayurvedic doctors often made medicines from local herbs. Patients seemed comfortable mixing their remedies and using whatever they perceived to be effective.

It is not ideology, then, that obstructs the use of modern curative medicine in rural Nepal, as much as the institutionalized way that government health services are delivered, which is alien to villagers. Traditional healers are part of the local community, whereas most government health workers come from urban areas outside the community and have a higher social status. Some health post staff managed to develop good rapport with local villagers, but many did not. Disenchanted with the isolation and discomforts of rural life, they were more interested in finding a way to transfer out. Their training usually had not included experience in rural areas or techniques for encouraging community involvement. For that matter, the ICHP practice of transferring staff frequently prevented strong ties between the community and health workers. This practice directly contradicted the primary health care philosophy of encouraging involvement in the local community.

Social division often contributed to patients' reluctance to utilize health services. Although villagers were encouraged by VHWs to seek treatment at health posts, they were often met with indifference when they followed this advice, owing to the social distance between patients and staff. Villagers were often reluctant to be treated by health workers who were young. Age commands respect in Nepal, but most health post staff were in their twenties because few older rural Nepalis could meet ICHP educational requirements. Administrative and staffing problems also discouraged villagers from seeking treatment at the posts. Sometimes treatment simply was not available because of the chronic shortages of medical supplies or because trained staff were frequently away from the posts when patients arrived.

Villagers were aware of their health problems, but when questioned many gave priority to health care for their agricultural animals. Though they were grieved by the frequent deaths of infants and children, they could always hope that another child would come. But it was almost impossible for poor farmers to find the money to replace a buffalo, on which the family's subsistence depended. Health post workers confirmed that villagers frequently asked for advice and medicine for their animals. Lalitpur's community health program, supported by United Mission to Nepal, sought to address this need directly by hiring a veterinarian to train its health workers in simple veterinary techniques. Government veterinary services were available only at the district level and not in all districts.

Despite their general willingness to use modern curative medicine, especially drugs, injections, and treatment for wounds, most villagers made no demand for modern preventive medicine. In fact, many misunderstood preventive measures. Men objected to vasectomy for fear that it would make them weak. Villagers were reluctant to give blood samples for the same reason. During visits I made to villagers' homes following an immunization campaign, women reported that they had avoided tetanus inoculation because it would prevent pregnancy. In one region, VHWs could not measure children's arm circumference to check for malnutrition because women feared the procedure would cause chicken pox; a chicken-pox epidemic had occurred in the area shortly after measuring began. To show a child's nutritional status, the tape measure was divided into three colors. Red indicated serious malnutrition; yellow, undernutrition; and green, adequate nourishment. Villagers in some areas said that if a child's arm measured in the red portion of the tape, it would die; if in the green, the stool would turn green and the child would die; if in the yellow, the child would get jaundice. Some villagers resisted using fluids—*nun-chini-paani* (salt-sugar-water) or RD Sol (a rehydration solution)—for diarrhea, since this treatment conflicts with the local practice of withholding fluids.

The District Health Office

According to ICHP plans, health activities at the district level were to be coordinated and supervised by the district health office and headed by a health inspector. The health inspector reported to the district medical officer, who was a medical doctor in charge of the district hospital. In reality, most health inspectors had little contact with the district medical officers, who had many other responsibilities in addition to their role in ICHP. Since none of the health inspectors were medical doctors themselves—many were former workers transferred from the malaria program— ICHP supervision from the district level was primarily administrative rather than medical.

The district health office had an important role to play both in providing support and supervision for health posts and in providing the link between the local and central levels. Yet district health officers did not exist in many areas, and existing offices were often understaffed. In 1978 only forty-eight of the seventy-five districts had district health offices, and only about 50 percent of these had a health inspector at work. Some had only a clerk, whose main responsibility was to compile statistics from the health posts and to convey these to the Ministry of Health in Kathmandu. Statistics were the primary form of information transmitted from the districts to health planners.

Like the Tate and Chittre health posts, the District I and II health offices differed markedly in staff size. The District I office had only a health inspector, a clerk/accountant, and a peon. It was in a new town, recently created by the government to replace the former district headquarters located in the hills. Government offices lined the town's only street, but houses were scarce, and as yet there was no water or electricity. Health workers willing to live under these conditions were hard to find. The health center, staffed by a health assistant and an ANM, was supported by neither a district hospital nor a district medical officer, although a fifteen-bed hospital was planned. One small shop sold a few drugs. Although the health center was a referral center for the health posts, it offered little more than a health post, except for a drug supply that was three times larger (funded by 18,000 rupees per year as compared with 6,000 rupees for each health post). In 1979, District I had eighteen health posts, of which three were unstaffed. It also had three Ayurvedic clinics, which were separately administered under the Department of Health Services in Kathmandu, bypassing the district medical officer and health inspector.

District I's health inspector had been transferred from the malaria program. He managed the district health office and supervised the health posts on periodic visits. Since there was no district medical officer, the inspector reported to the chief district officer for administration and to the Department of Health Services in Kathmandu. His job was difficult, since he had to visit all eighteen health posts. He described these visits as "just running": "In fifteen days, I am able to visit three to four health posts. I only stop to talk, then go on." It takes several days to walk between posts in remote areas. He recently had visited six health posts with a Kathmandu doctor to conduct vasectomy camps. To get any action on his requests required a trip to Kathmandu. I met him there frequently getting supplies and arranging for vasectomy camps.

Few foreigners had visited District I, according to the inspector; most stayed in Kathmandu. He wanted District I selected as a pilot district for the new nutrition program so that he could have more direct contact with UNICEF, which was supporting nutrition activities, and could obtain more supplies and equipment. The work done in the district office consisted mainly of tabulating statistics and preparing reports.

By contrast, District II's health office was located in the busy compound of the zonal hospital. This district health office was headed by the district medical officer, a medical doctor, who divided his time between the hospital, the outpatient clinic, and the district health office. He was one of only two medical officers I met who were actively involved in ICHP. He estimated that he spent one half-hour daily on the integrated program. Even such limited direction made this district health office unique, because of the medical officer's leadership, his understanding of the program, and his grasp of local conditions.

Sixteen of the nineteen staff positions in the district health office were filled in March 1979: district public health officer, health inspector, assistant health inspector, senior assistant health worker, family planning assistant, assistant health educator, laboratory technician, public health nurse, senior malaria assistant, statistics assistant, health education technician, laboratory assistant (two), assistant nurse-midwife, assistant health worker, accountant, clerk, and peons (two). Many of the staff were on leave or in the field, however, and others were working on statistical reports.

Field supervision was more feasible in District II, with its large staff, than in District I, where the health inspector was alone. According to the health post workers, the District II health inspector had provided them with regular and useful supervision, but he was on a two-year study leave in the United States, financed by USAID, and had not been replaced. The assistant health inspector visited the health posts in his place, but not as often. The malaria and family planning assistants also made field visits. Leprosy surveillance was supervised by the Leprosy Mission.

The district medical officer discussed his problems: the center (the Ministry of Health in Kathmandu) frequently ordered personnel transfers without consulting the district, and communicating with the center, even though facilitated by phone, mail service, road, and plane, was difficult. He rarely received a response to his letters. He described the ICHP administration as rigid. For example, recently he had written to the center saying that the immunization program could not be conducted year-round because of rains and the malaria-transmission season. The center replied that the program must be the same in all districts, and so it must be conducted throughout the year. This doctor was invited to all meetings in Kathmandu and was popular with visiting foreign health personnel. He had a prestigious family background and influential personal and professional connections. Even so, it was difficult for him to make changes that would adapt the health program to local conditions.

Problematic Roles of Health Workers

The Invisible Health Worker: The Peon[3]

The idea that peons, the "gofers" of the Nepali bureaucracy, provided health services may seem incongruous. But, in fact, during my visits to health posts not only in Tate and Chittre but in several other parts of Nepal, including Kathmandu Valley, a pattern emerged. After walking several hours to reach a health post, I frequently arrived, just as patients do, to find the trained health worker away—sometimes for a day, more often for several—supervising VHWs in the field, on official business in the district or center, or on personal leave. The peon remained at the post alone, informally interviewing and diagnosing patients, though he was not supposed to distribute medicine in the health assistant's absence. In each of the twenty-four health posts and ten hospitals I visited, I found peons actively involved in health care, and in nine cases the peon was the only health worker available. A health inspector in western Nepal reported in September 1978 that three of the eight health posts in his district had trained health workers; the other five were staffed only by peons.

Peons also interacted with patients when the trained health workers were present. In many posts they worked with the health assistants, dispensing medicines and telling patients how to use them, giving injections, and dressing wounds. After clinic hours, patients would go to the peon's home for emergencies. Peons treated patients not only at remote, understaffed posts but also in fully integrated centers with a complete staff of health assistants, assistant health workers, and assistant nurse-midwives. At one health post in Kathmandu Valley, which at the time of my visit had a visiting doctor conducting a tuberculosis clinic, a fully trained supervisory nurse, one foreign nurse seeing maternal and child health patients, a nutrition assistant, several paramedicals, and a peon, a farmer arrived with a severely bleeding cut from an axe wound. There was considerable stir among the other patients to make room for this emergency. The staff merely glanced up from their work as the peon seated the patient, applied pressure to stop the bleeding, dressed the wound, and arranged to have the patient transported to the nearest district hospital.

In Bir Hospital, Kathmandu's main government hospital, patients in the emergency room and outpatient clinics often relied on the peons to explain what the doctors said to them or to tell them where to go after being seen by the doctor for medicine, X-rays, or follow-up clinics. Peons functioned as cultural interpreters for the patients, many of whom were confused and intimidated by the hospital routine and by the doctors, who rarely spoke directly to patients to explain their condition or treatment. Thus, the peon not only was the most available staff person in rural health posts but was frequently the person who had the most interaction with patients in hospitals.

On further investigation, it became clear that the peon was the only real local worker in the health program. He lived in the village, spoke the local dialect, and knew the patients and their families. Villagers did not sense a status differential with peons, as they did with the health assistants, who were usually educated urbanites from Kathmandu with sophisticated clothing and manners. The peon was always available, either at the post or in the village, whereas the trained workers were away from the post much of the time. As noted earlier, most health assistants were unfamiliar with rural conditions and local dialects. Many were unhappy about being assigned to remote areas away from family and friends and modern amenities. Since health assistants were transferred frequently, they had little opportunity or desire to become part of the local community.

The peon was generally from a local farming family and took the job for the cash income, as the example of the Tate peon demonstrates. Although within the government hierarchy the peon's job had the lowest status, for many villagers any government job had a high status, especially since jobs were scarce in rural areas. Most peons were illiterate or had only a little education, and consequently they were ineligible for government jobs above the menial level. Although they had no formal health training, they learned to diagnose patients' symptoms, give injections, and apply dressings either from observation or from the health assistant's instruction.

My inquiry into peons' activities did not attempt to evaluate the effectiveness of their services but to describe their availability, accessibility, and willingness to provide some of the services villagers wanted. District health inspectors and district doctors reported that many peons were doing their job well, especially those who had good training and supervision from health assistants. One district doctor in eastern Nepal commented that the peon there, although not formally trained, had worked at the hospital for twenty-seven years and had more experience than the doctor. During my four days of observation at this hospital, there were always many more patients waiting to see the peon than the doctor.

What motivates the peon to perform tasks that are beyond his job description and training, when his salary is so meager? His government job and informally acquired skills do raise the peon's status in his community. Even without education or training, the peon is often seen as more skillful than a village health worker, who has very low status because he is unable to treat patients or distribute medicine. The peon is often older than the other health workers, which also raises his status, although villagers respect anyone with education (such as the health assistant). The peon provides services that villagers define as most needed—first aid, medicines, and injections. For villagers, the peon is not invisible. In fact, for many, he represents their only access to the government medical system.

Since the peon has no opportunity for promotion, he is not transferred and remains at home. He has few links with the district and central levels and no need to be away from the post to lobby at these levels for advancement. He has a strong base and support in the community and relies upon the patronage of the panchayat, which hires him. Therefore, he remains the one health worker over whom the community has some control.

For the trained health workers, who usually come from

outside the area, the peon is a valuable resource, able to provide information about the village and access to local elites. In addition, he does many of the more routine jobs that they do not like. His presence also frees the trained workers for other tasks and allows them to spend time away from the health post.

In my talks with health officials in Kathmandu, most denied that peons could actually be treating patients. The peon's job description and lack of formal training both argued against this role. The officials responded lightly or incredulously to my reports and inquiries about the peon's participation in health care delivery. It became a joke among some foreign advisors and Nepali officials that I was studying the role of the peon in Nepal's health service. But some of the most senior health officers, those with considerable field experience, confirmed my observations. Others who knew about the situation often denied the peon's role, for it departed from policy and confirmed reports that health workers were not doing the jobs for which they had been trained.

The WHO consultant on community participation responded to my description of the peon's activities by saying that peons should provide courier and custodial services and nothing more. Once the health post staffs were strengthened, peons would not need to do other tasks. He maintained that they had no role in community participation and might in fact be threatened by the training of volunteers, which would diminish their prestige.

Why does the peon remain invisible, his role in the delivery of health services unrecognized? The structure and practices of government and foreign bureaucracies are part of the reason. Foreign advisors and planners often do not know how peons are functioning because they are too busy to visit rural health posts. They regard peons as servants whose role does not merit serious consideration in policymaking and planning. Nepali bureaucrats also fail to recognize the peons' contribution, perhaps because of the South Asian "cultural blindness" toward untrained workers who perform menial or dirty tasks. Although peons are the most numerous employees of the Ministry of Health, this position was not evaluated in the midterm review of the health services (1979), which covered all other categories of employees. Nor was "peon" listed as a category in the Health Manpower Survey in June 1980.

Even when planners were told about the peon, they tended to disregard the information. They did not investigate its relevance to the proposed community health volunteer program or explore what could be learned from studying who peons are and what motivates them to acquire skills and give health services. One reason for the planners' indifference could be that to recognize that a local health worker similar to the Chinese "barefoot doctor" is already in place could make their own work more difficult.

International health organizations come to Nepal, as well as to other countries, with policy guidelines that they are committed to follow. Once a policy direction has been set in Geneva or Washington, planners in Kathmandu have no mechanism for adjusting it. Planners need to create new programs to appropriate allocated money, which must be spent in order to justify the mission of the organization. One of the best ways to spend funds is by organizing workshops and training programs that employ both foreigners and Nepalis. The kind of apprentice training that peons now receive is not susceptible to the kinds of training programs with which planners are familiar.

Thus, at a time when the Kathmandu health bureaucracy was preoccupied with how to obtain community participation and develop a community health volunteer to provide basic health services, no one was looking at the only existing truly community-based health worker. Planning discussions dealt with whom to recruit, what responsibilities to assign, and how to train, and reflected unfamiliarity with local conditions and the local political structure. I told planners about peons' activities not to advocate the formalization of their status as community health workers but to demonstrate the importance of understanding what happens at the local level. The case of the peon illustrates how the momentum of international policy can obscure the realities at the delivery level. Programs may reflect the organizational demands of the funding agencies and the values and culture of the planning bureaucracies more than the culture of the recipients.

I have reservations about calling attention to the peon for fear that if his contributions were recognized, his position might be reevaluated and formalized. Peons might then receive training and become part of the promotional hierarchy, removing them from the villages and undermining their present effectiveness. At the moment, they remain invisible and effective.

The Community Health Volunteer and the Village Health Worker

While planners in Kathmandu continued to debate the role of community health volunteers, training had begun in selected districts, including District I and District II. Two months prior to my visit, the Chittre health assistant and a health educator from District II had conducted a two-day training session in Chittre for health coordinators and volunteers, which several panchayat council members attended. The health coordinators were panchayat leaders who would select and help supervise the volunteers. A small per diem payment was given to volunteers for attending the training sessions, and members of elite families often participated.

Five coordinators whom I interviewed described the training as useful, especially the sections on health education and first aid. A twenty-year-old female volunteer, a daughter of Chittre's panchayat member, giggled when I asked her about her training and responsibilities. She had learned of her selection by a letter from the health post requesting that she serve as a volunteer and come to the training session. At the session, where participants received twenty rupees each, Nepali was spoken, but she spoke only Gurung, and consequently her comprehension was limited. She explained that she was required to give lessons about rehydration fluid, to help with deliveries or contact the ANM if needed, to encourage people to go to the health post or to the zonal hospital when sick, and to teach about *charphis* (latrines) and safe drinking water. She did not visit homes, but she talked to women when they went for water or got together at night; she added that the women forgot the things she told them. She did not know who the health coordinators were in her area. Our visit was the first time she had met the village health worker.

In District I, training sessions for health coordinators, conducted by the health inspector, began in April 1979. The participants, who were elite rural leaders, had difficulty understanding many parts of the community health volunteer manual. As in Chittre, village coordinators and volunteers agreed that they found the first aid training the most useful. Villagers confirmed that they needed simple first aid treatment and criticized the village health workers for being unable to provide it. Although they received first aid instruction, community health volunteers were not given any supplies or medicines, a fact that severely limited their ability to meet village expectations. The health post peon often had higher status in villagers' eyes, since he had access to the limited health post supplies. The job description for community health volunteers overlapped with that for village health workers. Both were performing primarily educational and motivational tasks, yet the volunteer was expected to work without pay, while the VHW was a paid staff member.

The VHW's job description required him to meet as many family members as possible during home visits to determine whether anyone had fever (malaria). If so, he took a blood slide and gave malaria medication. He examined rashes for possible smallpox, checked persistent coughs for tuberculosis, and watched for any signs of leprosy or other illnesses. He referred suspected cases to the health post for treatment and followed up on any previously diagnosed cases. In the area of maternal and child health, he inquired about sick children, measured the arms of children under five, and taught about the use of *sarbottom pitho* (fortified flour) for those who were undernourished and *nun-chini-paani* (salt-sugar-water for rehydration) for infants with diarrhea. He encouraged pregnant women to go to the health post and advised mothers to have their children immunized; he identified and motivated eligible couples for family planning and sterilization; and he provided general health education and motivated families to go to the health post. (See Appendix 3 for full job description.)

Some village health workers were receiving limited supplies of drugs to distribute, even though they were not always adequately trained for this responsibility. VHWs in District II received their first supply of drugs during field visits in 1979, though no instructions for diagnosis and distribution were given. They had one tube of eyedrops, ten aspirin tablets, and eighty worm pills for the month. In District I, the health inspector did not give these to the VHWs but used them to supplement the health post supply, asking how the VHWs could treat patients' needs with only one pill or one eyedrop. In another district, the VHW combined all varieties of pills in one bag. He distributed these to patients, carefully recording the date and quantity given, without understanding that different pills were appropriate for different symptoms.

Few officials at the central level understood the difficulty of the village health worker's role. My own observation confirmed that physical limitations alone made it nearly impossible for the VHWs to perform the many tasks outlined. Yet discussions on VHWs during planning sessions for the next development plan focused on how to increase their responsibilities, including their supervision of community health volunteers. The representatives from the vertical health projects contributed suggestions for additional tasks for these workers which would better cover the priorities of each project. There seemed to be no concern for evaluating the limited feasibility of the VHW's present assignment.

The VHW program provides an excellent example of an opportunity for coordination between donor agencies. USAID and Health Associates were working with the ICHP Training Division to develop a new VHW job description. At the same time, Britain Nepal Medical Trust, through contact with health post staff in connection with their tuberculosis program, were aware of the VHW's problems and had informally begun working with VHWs to develop a better training and supervision program in Sankhuwasabha District. While visiting health posts in eastern Nepal, I was impressed with the effect this support had on the VHWs' work and told the USAID representative and advisors about it. As a result, a meeting was arranged and plans were proposed to coordinate ICHP, USAID, and Britain Nepal Medical Trust's training for VHWs. Although small voluntary and mission programs have their disadvantages, my field observation indicated that the personnel in these groups, because they work at the grass roots, were frequently more sensitive to the social and cultural aspects of delivering health services.

In meetings sponsored by the Department of Health Services to encourage community participation, such as the conference described in chapter three, discussions focused on who to recruit as community health volunteers, what responsibilities to assign them, and how to train villagers to carry out these responsibilities. Various proposals were put forward, but they all reflected unfamiliarity with local conditions and with the local political structure. It was this preoccupation with establishing a program of community health volunteers that made me give more serious consideration to how work is allocated at health posts and to the identification of the real community workers—the peons.

The roles of village health workers, community volunteers, and peons illustrate the resistance of bureaucracy to information that may otherwise be widely recognized. Village health workers had been assigned impossible tasks, which they could not manage to do, yet policy regarding their activities was not being changed. The same mistake was being repeated in the case of community health volunteers (as described in chapter three). Peons at health posts, paid for custodial work, were providing essential health services that remained unacknowledged. In each case the failure to give adequate attention to local conditions produced unexpected results at the local level.

My tour of health posts had uncovered several pervasive problems that all were struggling with to some degree. Many health post staff members had difficulty adjusting to rural areas because of their urban social and cultural backgrounds. Usually their training had not prepared them for the working conditions. As a result, their morale was often poor, their ties to the community were weak, and they did not communicate effectively with their patients. Ethnic and language differences within rural areas made communication more difficult.

Some jobs at health posts were difficult or impossible to carry out, because job descriptions designed in Kathmandu were unrealistic in light of local conditions. Links with the local community, through the panchayats and health committees, were tenuous, as were links with Kathmandu, through the district health offices. Thus, support and supervision from the local and district levels were erratic at best. Shortages of resources, especially drugs and other supplies, thwarted efforts to provide care.

Despite those difficulties, in some ways ICHP was working at the village level as planned. The conscientious health assistant at Tate had established a good rapport with the local community and was providing health services, even though the lack of supplies and district support made his job difficult. In Chittre, similarly, some of the staff were working effectively, though their efforts, too, were hindered by limited resources.

In other ways, ICHP was not working. Village health workers could not complete their rounds, they provided few effective services, and they were poorly regarded by the community. Many posts were not coping as well as Tate and Chittre with the problems of delivering services, often because staff morale was too poor to surmount the difficulties.

In still other ways, ICHP was working, but not at all as planned. The training provided to health assistants often filtered down unexpectedly to peons, who, after serving an informal apprenticeship, were well placed by their availability and close community ties to provide effective health services, drawing on the resources of the post.

5

Sources and Channels of Information

Planners need different kinds of information about the recipient country at different stages of planning. In addition to information on local administrative procedures and economic resources, they may need only general information about the local culture to formulate an overall policy on financial assistance and project guidelines. But the closer the plans are to the actual delivery of services, the greater the need for detailed cultural information.

The officials I interviewed in the donor agencies and in the government generally agreed that cultural information is rarely used in planning. Among several reasons they gave, the most important were that cultural information was not available or accessible and that when it was available, it was not very useful.

The main sources of information for planners were reports prepared by donor agencies and the government; personal experience, including field travel; and exchange through formal and informal meetings. But the sources of information are only the beginning of the story—how information is transmitted is equally important. By examining the flow of information, it is possible to see how the structure and demands of the planning bureaucracies have determined what information is available to planners and how useful they perceive it to be.

Sources of Information

Reports

Government and donor agencies produce many kinds of reports, often voluminous: background papers, feasibility studies, annual reports, progress evaluations, and project proposals. Donor agency staff in Nepal spend much of their time preparing reports for the regional office or for their headquarters in Europe or North America. They write in their offices in Kathmandu, using information gathered chiefly from official government policy statements and reports and from conversations with relevant Nepali officials.

What information staff members use in reports depends on agency procedures, however, which do not always allow for an accurate portrayal of local conditions. For example, in 1978 one multinational agency gave assistance to ten projects in Nepal. Its staff in Kathmandu was expected to work with Nepali counterparts to prepare a general document outlining the agency's agreements with the government covering the projects, as well as separate documents for each project. The agency coordinator said that he actually was writing the reports himself and that he tried to make the documents as realistic as possible by describing the working situation in Nepal, but that he was limited in what and how he wrote because he had to follow a given format. This rigid format was difficult to adapt to individual countries because it required detailed plans to fit agency policy and made no allowances for the differing local structures and rhythms of life in recipient countries. The coordinator described the format as superimposing the agency's own structure on Nepal's needs. In his view, the agency's highest priorities were that the program be financially sound and show quick results.

The headquarters of donor agencies usually provide policy guidelines along with funding. According to official procedure, the agency representatives in Nepal, in consultation with government officials, identify broad areas of need that fall within these guidelines and submit a written proposal of a general plan to headquarters. The headquarters then sends out consultants or reconnaissance missions to evaluate the plan. After meeting with various officials, the consultants write reports with their recommendations. Next, a new set of agency staff and/or consultants write feasibility studies and project proposals. After specific projects are funded, the local agency staff submit biannual or annual reports to headquarters describing progress and making recommendations for extension or for additional funding.

Despite the agency commitment to consultation with government officials, Nepalis often participate little in this process. A former USAID advisor cynically described what he called "collaborative style": "The content of USAID's project paper is determined by the U.S. Congress. The basic papers are then written by USAID staff without Nepali input; instead, the country office brings in consultants with special skills to write each section of the report. All this data is of interest only to the agency."

Additional reports may be demanded. For example, to supplement its annual and project reports, the United Nations Fund for Population Activities (UNFPA) decided to have a "needs assessment report for population" prepared in Spring 1979 by a team of six foreign consultants (UNFPA 1978). Altogether, the report was six months in preparation. Before the consultants arrived in Nepal, the UNFPA representative tried to put together all available quantifiable data (UNFPA 1979). He hired two local consultants—a resident American anthropologist and a Nepali statistician—to inventory population-related social research (Cardinalli 1979) and data on the health-delivery system (Chowdhari 1979). On arriving, the team interviewed government officials and workers in other agencies on their activities in areas related to population. They read government plans for the next five to seven years and projected resources needed to carry out these plans. They reviewed results from earlier programs and gaps in current and future programs. The team produced an extensive report incorporating the background data and its own observations and recommendations (Sikkel 1979). Since then, additional teams of consultants have been sent to Nepal to spend one to two months assessing areas recommended for funding—women and development, health services, and so on. Each team also writes a report on its activities, findings, and recommendations.

The timing of donor agency reports is almost always determined by the agency's yearly budget cycle and not by Nepal's planning cycle. For example, in 1978–79 the USAID country office was preparing its proposal for assistance to Nepal's health programs. In order to meet the USAID deadline, this proposal had to be submitted to Washington before the Nepal government had determined its health priorities for the 1980–85 five-year development plan. The AID health officer arranged meetings with the Secretary of Health, the Director General of Health Services, the Planning Unit, chiefs of the vertical health projects, and the chief of ICHP to discuss the government's priorities for assistance from AID. The Nepali officials did not formulate specific requests; instead, they asked the AID officer to describe a project to which they could respond. Thus, because of USAID's schedule, USAID's Nepal staff was forced to formulate plans that might not agree with the Ministry of Health's official programs.

Producing reports on schedule is a high priority in the agencies, and one that can consume much of the staff's energy. Agency staff and advisors tend to work against deadlines. They are inaccessible for weeks when under pressure to complete reports. Most agencies expect their staff to write their own reports, even if another agency has already provided good coverage on the same topic. The justification given by the agencies for this duplication of effort is that each has its own organizational requirements and must have special reports to meet them.[1]

But there is also the difficulty of finding out what others have done. In 1979 neither Nepal nor WHO had a central library for documents on health. Thus, to know what documentation was available and where it could be obtained was a big problem. Some reports are kept by government departments and/or by donor agencies in Kathmandu, but many older reports are available only in donor agency headquarters in Washington, Geneva, or elsewhere. For example, Health Associates kept an extensive library on Nepal in its New York office. One learns about such reports either by chance or through extensive searching and perseverance. I had to visit each government department and individual agency to assemble my collection. As a result, there were times when I had copies of relevant reports that were unknown or inaccessible to planners and administrators. I probably had one of the most complete sets available anywhere at that time. Consultants and advisors, especially those assigned to Kathmandu for a short period, cannot be expected to follow this same time-consuming procedure to gather information. The simple procedure of depositing one copy of every report made by any agency in the library at Tribhuvan University in Nepal would be one way to offset the failure of collective memory.

The same exercises, producing similar reports, are repeated year after year. One agency representative, who had a shelf of reports on Nepal, commented that they were produced by various agencies and government departments without any follow-up. He said that such reports usually reflected a compromise between agency and country politics and were therefore superficial and unsatisfactory. Thus, he rarely used them. He also had several books and various documents sent by UNFPA, Economic and Social Commission of Asia and the Pacific (ESCAP), the Population Institute, and WHO, but he said that he rarely used these either, because he had no time for reading books.

The foreign planners and administrators therefore spend an enormous amount of time writing reports that they expect to be disregarded. It is doubtful whether Nepali officials consider surveys and reports useful either. The Project Formulation for ICHP (Nepal Department of Health Services 1976), a lengthy exercise, was funded by foreign assistance and made heavy use of foreign consultants. It has never been signed by the government and thus is not official, but Nepali administrators referred to it when asked about the components of ICHP. At the same time, they implied that such cumbersome plans presented only the ideal.

A Nepali administrator in ICHP said that he used the program's numerous reports to provide data to the endless stream of foreigners who came to see him, not because of the quality or accuracy of the reports, but because he wanted all visitors to use the same sources so that they would be working with the same statistics. This strategy also reduced the time he had to spend with the foreigners, who asked many of the same questions. A senior Nepali health official, commenting on the Nepal Country Health Profile (World Health Organization 1979), which took foreign consultants and government officials several years to prepare, said: "This report is for others [meaning foreigners], as the Nepalis know what is in it already." Another official said that in Nepal information is exchanged orally. Even with modern bureaucratic procedures, people obtain more information by speaking to each other than by reading reports.

Many reports included social and cultural information, often in the introductory and background sections. Agencies such as UNFPA and USAID hired social scientists to write the "social soundness analysis": an assessment of the sociocultural feasibility of a project, its likely social impact on different groups, and the potential "spread effect" of the practices and institutions to be introduced. Judging by the documents themselves, there is little evidence that such information actually influenced the final recommendations for donor assistance. In USAID's project paper outlining its aid to Nepal's health and family planning programs, the "social soundness analysis" was condensed to three pages in the body of the report and eight in the annex (USAID 1980:14–17; Annex G:1–8). Agency representatives whom I interviewed implied that it was included primarily as a formality to fulfill the requirements specified by Congress. A WHO staff member in the South-East Asia Regional Office responded to reports containing descriptive sociocultural information by asking why social scientists had to write such long reports and include "everything." The final report edited by the regional office deleted much of the descriptive material but retained the numbers.

Field Travel

Senior officials and consultants from the headquarters of donor agencies get some information on visits to recipient countries, which are made partly for reasons of protocol but also to supplement reports received from field representatives. In Nepal the timing of the visits often coincided with the pleasant weather and with the agency's yearly work cycle. Hosting these visits could be a very time-consuming responsibility for the agency staff residing in the country. Generally, the visitors also met with high-level government officials in formal settings in the capital.

Sometimes agency representatives living in Nepal supplemented their Kathmandu sources of information by making field visits, perhaps accompanied by government officials or colleagues from other agencies. I asked agency representatives and Nepali officials how many and what kind of field visits they had made during their assignment in Nepal. The majority, including Nepalis, said that their experience outside Kathmandu was too limited. Although several indicated that they would like to make field visits, their responsibilities in Kathmandu and the difficulty of travel kept them from broadening their understanding of rural Nepal.

Since most rural areas can be reached only on foot, and many are inaccessible for many months of the year, most field visits are made during the dry months. Officials therefore remain unaware of the difficult conditions experienced by both patients and health workers during the monsoon season. Travel by vehicles, when possible, is likely to be uncomfortable. Even plane travel in the mountains can be precarious, and flights are frequently canceled. Lodging and food, where available, are often viewed by officials as inadequate. It is necessary when visiting rural areas to carry sleeping equipment and food, as I did when visiting health posts. Foreigners, especially, worry about unhygienic conditions. Planned field excursions are often canceled because of such difficulties and because of the time constraints imposed by responsibilities in Kathmandu.

As a result, a few accessible health facilities are frequently visited, while most are never visited at all. Some health posts located on motorable roads are visited so often that they have guest books containing the names of such important persons as the director of WHO, the regional director of UN-ICEF, and the Minister of Health. Health posts along the Pokhara road or near Pokhara, one of the largest valleys in Nepal and a favorite tourist spot, are among those most often visited, since the road and accommodations are good. The trip from Kathmandu to Pokhara can be made in a day, even with stops to inspect health facilities on the way, and one can fly back, leaving junior staff to return in the jeep. Often visitors travel in a caravan of two or three vehicles, showing little awareness of the overwhelming impact the arrival of several foreign and senior personnel has on the health post staff, the patients, and the surrounding community.

The health facilities easily accessible by road are often not typical of those in more remote areas. They are generally better staffed and better equipped, since transport is available to bring supplies and supervision from the capital. Staff are more willing to remain there, since they can more easily travel to urban areas to visit their families or strengthen professional ties. These facilities are also more accessible to patients and therefore tend to have higher attendance at clinics. Finally, these facilities have better means of communication. Kathmandu officials can easily notify them about scheduled visits, ensuring that the staff will be present when visits occur and allowing the staff to prepare the premises for inspection.

By visiting only model health posts, foreign advisors and Nepali officials receive the impression that the rural health program is functioning according to plan. They do not learn that most health posts are understaffed, poorly equipped and supplied, and poorly supervised. When remote health centers are visited, it is only sporadically and briefly. Helicopters make it possible to reach hill and mountain regions, but visits usually last only an hour or two because these trips typically cost some $600 per hour. Officials I interviewed recognized the limitations of such short inspections but defended their usefulness.[2]

Not all donor agency representatives considered site visits

essential. Some said that they did not need to visit rural areas in Nepal because they had had experience in other developing countries. A frequently heard saying is that "all villages in Third World countries are the same."

Formal and Informal Meetings

Personal interaction is a third source of information, but it too is limited in range. Not only do foreigners visit the same few rural health facilities time and again; they also meet the same Nepali government officials time and again when they are in Kathmandu. These are Nepalis in senior positions who speak English and are accustomed to meeting Westerners. Some foreign advisors study and speak Nepali, depending on the length of their assignment in Nepal and their interest in the language, but not many feel comfortable using Nepali in official settings, especially when their government counterparts speak English fluently. Certain Nepali officials are identified by foreign advisors as being responsive to their needs, and they are the ones who are contacted most often by the advisors and who appear most frequently at informal social gatherings.

Kathmandu hosts a large number of representatives from bilateral, multilateral, and private voluntary organizations. Not only does each donor agency come with its own policy and programs, but its representatives come with assumptions grounded in their national culture which determine their styles of interaction. The differences can result in confusion and culture conflict. Nepali health officials are confronted with Germans, Swiss, Japanese, Canadians, and Americans connected with bilateral agencies; the French coordinator of WHO programs; the Norwegian representative from UNICEF; the British representative from the private agency Save the Children; and the Americans from the Dooley Foundation and so on. An interview I had with the Nepali coordinator of several rural development projects, who was educated in the United States and popular with Westerners, was interrupted by three unscheduled foreign visitors, a Nepali researcher, and six phone calls from donor agencies requesting appointments or setting up conferences, all within one hour. I observed the contrasting ways in which these individuals presented their requests, and the coordinator's skill at adapting to the rapid changes in styles of interaction.

Most meetings dealing with specific projects take place in government offices in the foreign aid section of the Ministry of Finance and the Ministry of Health and the Department of Health Services. From observing and talking to agency advisors, I gained the impression that meetings are requested by the donor agencies more often than by the Nepal government. Considerable time is spent in arranging and holding meetings. This was especially true in ICHP, because the project chief was frequently away attending international meetings (sponsored by the donor agencies) and was very much in demand when he was in Kathmandu. Since he was the only person able to make any decision about ICHP, all donor representatives had to meet with him directly—and the number of donors, both large and small, was considerable. One representative from a private organization based in eastern Nepal experienced three broken appointments during a single week, a series of frustrations that did not seem to be unusual. Advisors frequently commented that they had not seen the chief for weeks or even months; some complained that their projects were stalled because they had not been able to see him.

Formal seminar meetings, usually organized and paid for by donor agencies, permit some exchange of information between Nepali officials and agency representatives. These meetings are used for such purposes as introducing new concepts and programs, coordinating the efforts of government and agency personnel in ICHP, and encouraging government officials to issue reports or policy statements.

More information is exchanged among donor representatives on an informal basis than in formal settings. Those assisting ICHP had regular breakfast meetings. They did not want any publicity about this arrangement for fear that senior government officials would oppose it, although they were unclear about why there would be opposition. Donor representatives living in Kathmandu have contact among themselves, but they have little contact with voluntary groups working and residing in rural areas, whose foreign personnel are more familiar with rural conditions and the problems of health care delivery.

In Kathmandu information is exchanged informally at social gatherings, such as the frequent receptions and dinners hosted by the international community. Many of these gatherings include Nepali counterparts and friends, but others are composed only of foreigners. Who attends and who talks to whom in this informal network are indications of status and influence. Foreigners compete for the special honor of having a senior government official, such as the Secretary of Health or a member of the Planning Commission, accept a social invitation.

Although there is a large number of foreigners in Kathmandu, the foreign community is small in the sense that most foreigners know each other personally or at least know about each other. Not only do foreigners tend to talk to the same Nepali officials but they also tend to talk to the same contacts within their own group. Often the conversation is directly work-related, incorporating rumors and gossip, which are a major form of communication in Kathmandu. It is difficult for foreigners to be part of the inner circle of the Nepal government, where contacts and decisions are often determined by kin relationships, and so it is frequently through rumors that they first learn of changes in government policy or personnel. Participants in the rumor network feel that they are part of what is going on.

The Nepal government channels information to the foreign community through *The Rising Nepal*, a local English-language newspaper. Most foreigners read it, because even those who speak Nepali fluently find the Devanagri script and journalistic language of the vernacular local papers difficult. *The Rising Nepal* is an official government paper, and it emphasizes events that explain and support government policy. When I asked one WHO advisor if he had any knowledge of a tradition of community participation in Nepal, his reply was that he believed there was a strong tradition in rural areas because every day he saw references to local development efforts in the newspaper. The government was encouraging community participation in all areas of development, not just health, and supported it by reporting successful local participation in building a road, providing a water supply, building a health post, and so on. The advisor was apparently unaware that in addition to reporting information, *The Rising Nepal* selects stories that emphasize successful efforts in support of government policy.

The Flow of Information within Government

Data, Plans, and Targets

Nepali planners work with some of the same limitations as their foreign counterparts. The officials appointed by the government to formulate long-term health plans in the early 1970s were often medical doctors, usually from Kathmandu, with limited rural experience and no formal planning experience. Members of the government teams explained that they obtained their information from government reports and relevant ministries and departments. Data obtained from field visits to rural health facilities were limited, since field travel presents the same obstacles for senior Nepali officials with urban backgrounds as for foreign consultants.

Among the three-member team appointed by the Palace in the Janch Bhuj Kendra (The Centre for Enquiry and Investigation) to formulate the long-term health plan in 1975, none had extensive experience in rural areas. Only one field trip outside Kathmandu was described. It was made by helicopter to Siklis, a large, wealthy Gurung village whose residents have the means to travel to the nearest urban area for medical care when needed, in contrast to many remote areas of Nepal, where people are dependent on local health services only. Rural experience was not tapped in writing the long-term health plan, even though the plan was intended to meet the national priorities established by the Palace and the expectations of the donor agencies—to extend minimum basic health services to the maximum number of people in rural areas.

Although government officials frequently said that foreigners do not understand local conditions and resources, many Nepali administrators and planners, because of their urban backgrounds and career positions in the Kathmandu administration, are also removed from the reality of rural conditions. Most officials rarely make field visits and do not see that information collected during such visits would be relevant to the planning procedure, which emphasizes quantitative data and targets.

The government's emphasis on setting and meeting targets largely determines what type of information on health status is collected. Targets are set for all activities of the Ministry of Health. In "Annual Targets of Center and Districts for Fiscal Year 2034/035 (1977/78)," issued by the government, only hospitals and Ayurvedic clinics lack specific targets. The country-wide targets for the Integrated Community Health Program that year were numerous:

> Establishment of 50 new integrated health posts and the conversion of old health posts to the integrated model; 60 *lakh* (one *lakh* equals 100,000) home visits by 898 village panchayat-based village health workers; construction of health post and district offices; to collect blood samples from 150,000 (10 percent) fever patients in fully integrated districts and treat positive cases found; number and category of health personnel and others to receive in-service training; to strengthen community health information system by putting into practice the various forms and registers of the information system in 292 health posts and district health offices; to strengthen the supervision project of 48 districts; to provide permanent sterilization to 4,000 married couples; to conduct nutrition surveillance, 700,000 times for three *lakh* children from 1 to 5 years of age; to immunize 75,000 children in integrated districts with DPT, BCG, and against smallpox.

Targets are set in accordance with the policy objectives provided by the Planning Commission and are transferred to the ministries concerned. The Ministry of Health then prepares its programs using the policy objectives, the targets, and the budget allocation. A member of the Planning Commission explained that once the ministry submits its five-year and annual plans, officials of the Ministry of Health and of the Planning Commission meet to ascertain whether the plans fit the government's overall objectives and priorities. Country-wide targets and budgets are then broken down into targets and budgets for the central and district levels; the district health office in turn divides its targets among the health posts. At the time of this research, district-level workers and those still farther down were not involved in preparing the annual plan.

Programs are evaluated by how well they meet their targets. The center must rely on statistical reports from its districts to determine whether targets have been met, thus structuring the type and flow of information from delivery level to the center. The system uses forms and registers for conveying this information.

In 1972, when the ICHP pilot projects were started, the program inherited 137 forms and registers (Nepal Department of Health Services 1977:19) from the vertical projects that were to be incorporated in ICHP. At that time, all reports had to be submitted to both the Department of Health Services and the vertical projects. By 1975, the number of forms had been reduced to forty-five by coordination with the chiefs of the vertical projects and advisory agencies. As described in the "Annual Report for 2034–35 (1977–78)," ICHP was able to develop a more efficient multipurpose system, which by 1979 was in various stages of implementation. There were twenty-two basic forms for recording the delivery of health services. Twelve forms and registers were used by all districts, at whatever stage of integration, for recording the services given by village health workers and the health post staff. Eleven additional forms and registers were used by fully integrated districts for records on malaria surveillance, treatment, and prevention. In addition, there were forms for special activities, such as the Expanded Program of Immunization, and administrative forms for the health post, including those for reporting on the annual drug supply, personnel matters, and financial transactions. Although the health information system relied on compiling data recorded on these forms, most forms were unavailable in 1978–79 because of a printing problem in Kathmandu. Health workers, therefore, were unable to record most statistics.

Vertical Barriers

Statistics recorded and transmitted from villages to the central government in Kathmandu show how targets structured the information system and influenced the functioning of health workers. As noted earlier, at the most remote level, collecting statistics was the job of the village health worker, who was expected to visit each house in his *vek* (local area) once a month (thirty houses a day). During each visit the VHW recorded information about the family in the village health register, indicating any illnesses, births, deaths, marriages, settlers, and new houses since the last visit. At the entrance of each house, he painted a stencil on which he recorded the dates of his visits. These were later checked by his supervisor, the health assistant. After twenty-seven days of visiting villages, the VHW returned to the health post for three nonsurveillance (reporting) days, so that the month's statistics from his village health register could be compiled and submitted.

In each district I visited, my research assistant and I accompanied at least one VHW on his rounds. Although there were some variations depending on the terrain and the layout of houses in the village, a basic pattern emerged. Generally we left the health post or VHW's residence after the morning meal of *daal bhaat* (rice and lentils) at about ten A.M. and walked for between a half-hour and two hours to reach the village to be surveyed that day. Our visits to the houses were brief because most were empty—during the day the men were working in the fields and the women were gathering wood and water or doing other domestic chores away from the house. At home were only older women and children, if anyone.

Most VHWs we accompanied attempted to perform their tasks conscientiously. They asked mainly about fever and sickness, attempted to measure the arms of any small children they encountered (although they did not seek children out), and told families about *aushadhi paani* (medicine water, which was the commonly used phrase for salt-sugar-water) if any diarrhea was reported. But at the majority of houses, the VHWs only dated and signed the stencil painted on the outside wall. In fact, we repeatedly heard villagers use the term *bhetta korne*, meaning "wall writer," in referring to VHWs. Asked to describe the VHWs' work, villagers replied that they only came and signed. They said that VHWs only occasionally asked whether anyone was sick or measured a child's arm.

Several times, villagers commented that our visit was the first time the VHW had told them about rehydration solution, general hygiene, family planning, and so forth. Most were unsure of our status, even though I explained that I was not with the Department of Health Services. Having spent time on this extra work, the VHW was unable to cover the thirty households required daily. Sometimes we were still in the village after six P.M., with a walk of an hour or two yet to be made in the dark.

The reality is that no one could carry out the VHW's prescribed responsibilities. Since the Department of Health Services emphasized covering all households in the *vek* and recording statistics in the register and on the house, VHWs gave these tasks high priority. This pattern conformed with the criteria used to evaluate VHWs. The health assistant whom we accompanied during field supervision only checked the stencils to see when the VHW had visited or asked villagers about whether the VHW had been there. There were few questions about what the VHW had asked or done. Thus, to meet the centrally established targets, VHWs had to carry out their responsibilities in this limited manner, even though the result did not provide the intended health services.

All statistics reported by VHWs at the end of the month were compiled by the health assistant and statistician (if there was one) and used in filling out forms showing the post's monthly attendance and morbidity and mortality rates. These rates, based on the health assistant's and

VHW's diagnoses made by clinical intuition or guesswork (Padfield 1978:11), were extremely unreliable. There was no indication that these statistics were being used by VHWs or health post workers to assess changes in community health status or to measure progress. The statistics were taken by the peon to the district health office, where they were compiled with statistics from other posts in the district and then forwarded to the statistics division of ICHP in Kathmandu. The statistician in ICHP explained that the district statistics were further compiled for quarterly and annual reports to the Ministry of Health and the Planning Commission, which compared the achievements to the targets originally set.

Prominently displayed in each health post and district health office was a large chart divided into monthly columns for the year, showing the total number of clinic and home visits made in the health post area. When inquiring about the type of services given in an area, I was always referred to these charts. A version of this chart showing the targets and statistics for all integrated districts hung in the ICHP office in Kathmandu. In response to my question about what information was useful, a senior health official turned and pointed to this chart, explaining that the program was evaluated and budgeted by comparing its achievements to the targets.

The importance of statistics was also reflected in staffing patterns. At the time of my research, district health offices were understaffed, especially those in the early phase of integration. In the districts I visited, even if there was no health inspector (the most senior post at this level), a statistician was often on duty. In some districts, such as Dhankuta and Sankhuwasabha, the statistician's position was the only one filled other than those of the clerks, and this staff administered the whole district program.

My observations of how data were being collected and recorded at the village and health post levels raised doubts about their accuracy and reliability. Administrators and planners in Kathmandu were also aware of this problem, but it did not seem to have primary importance for them. What was more important was the existence of statistical data that could be exchanged throughout the system to justify the functioning of the administration and to meet the expectations of the government and donor agencies. The use of recorded data at the collection base—that is, at the field level—did not appear to be an issue either.

The formal information system's function was largely restricted to transmitting statistical data. Since there were not substantive or situational reports from villages and health posts, the only means of communicating such information to higher levels of government was by letter or direct contact. But rural health workers in ICHP, sensitive to their low status and security, did not risk notice and possible criticism by writing other than what was required. Even more senior officers, who had access to the center because of personal status and kinship, were discouraged by the lack of response to their reports and requests. A senior official of ICHP encouraged district workers to visit him in Kathmandu. But on arriving, workers often found him too busy to meet them. Even if they did meet this official, they rarely felt that action was taken on the issues discussed. The evidence from my research is supported by the midterm health review (1979), which found that among health workers in the programs surveyed, those in ICHP had the lowest expectation of receiving any response to their reports.

Meetings and workshops held in Kathmandu were another way of getting information from the districts to the center. Although some of these meetings included field workers, they were generally limited to district-level doctors and health inspectors. The formal protocol of meetings and the presence of senior officials, such as the Minister of Health, could be intimidating to more junior participants.

A health inspector in a remote district commented to me on how useless he found these meetings and how frustrated he was by the center's inattention to suggestions and requests from rural workers:

> One of the biggest problems in Nepal is that people who are involved in implementation should be involved in planning. We only have workshops once a year. At these we can only discuss the way the plan is working—how to fulfill the targets. At these meetings, no one listens to people like village health workers because of their low status. The international

agencies sponsor conferences like the National Conference on Primary Health Care held last year and then issue reports. The organizations like UNICEF and USAID want publications as propaganda, but these don't change anything. Most senior officials, including the Minister, attend the opening sessions of these meetings and influential advisors to the Minister are present throughout the discussions, but these people don't listen to district-level people. In Nepal we have developed a tradition to get people to give suggestions, but then do nothing about them. Workshops are merely a way of spending money from aid. We have poor working conditions in rural areas, such as lack of supplies and staff which affect our efficiency, but no one at the Center is interested.

Many other rural workers echoed his remarks during my visits.

Some health inspectors in districts accessible to Kathmandu came to the center and used their personal connections to get the supplies they needed when there was no response to their written requests. Often these were the men who had formerly worked in the malaria project, which was better organized than ICHP and more responsive to the needs of its personnel. Because of their earlier experience, they still expected a response from central project administrators. But most health inspectors were too far away to afford time and money for such trips unless they were officially invited. Although the health inspector theoretically was responsible for the program's success in his district, the ICHP administration in Kathmandu appeared almost indifferent to whether health inspectors were actually on duty in the integrated districts. As mentioned earlier, in many districts the administration of ICHP was left to clerical staff because there was no inspector. When I was preparing for district visits, the central administration often referred me to the district health inspector, but several times I arrived in the district only to find that the inspector had been transferred a month or even a year before, or that he was away on extended leave or for other reasons. My experiences revealed a gap in the center's knowledge of district staffing and operations.

Center officials were supposed to make supervisory visits

to each district biannually, but they came only once a year, if at all. According to district and local health workers, these visits were rarely made for local problem solving and supervision. Almost always they were occasioned by special purposes—to host visiting foreigners, to prepare the way for the king's regional visit, to conduct training programs, to collect specific information requested by the Ministry of Health or another government office, and so on. Following the pattern of visits by donor agencies, the more easily accessible district centers and health posts were visited most frequently. Even the accessible districts were not necessarily visited regularly, however. In the Terai, where there is road access from Kathmandu and from the district centers to the health posts, two of the ICHP pilot districts reported that no one from the center had visited them for over three years.

Visits were not always used effectively for exchanging information. I accompanied one ICHP official and a foreign advisor on a supervisory visit to three districts in the Terai. This trip had a dual purpose: the ICHP official was gathering information required for the annual malaria evaluation, and the foreign advisor was testing new forms for district-level supervision. Most of our time was spent in each district reviewing the statistical reports. As one district doctor observed, this information could easily have been obtained from the monthly reports sent to Kathmandu, allowing time for the district staff to discuss other issues and problems with the visitors.

At the district level, health inspectors were also supposed to make supervisory visits to the health posts. But most inspectors, especially those from small, understaffed offices, did not make many field visits; as several said, there was no one else to run the office if they went away. Travel was again an obstacle, even in the Terai, where most areas are accessible by road. Health workers had difficulty obtaining government vehicles to use, and gasoline was scarce and expensive. The travel and daily allowances were very low, and the workers were generally not reimbursed for long periods, if at all. Inspectors therefore obtained most of their information about health post activities from the statistical reports brought into the district center at the end of the month. Most health workers in rural areas were originally from Kathmandu or the Terai and did not want to remain in remote and hill districts. Their efforts to communicate with Kathmandu were directed toward obtaining personal transfers, an activity that took much of their time and necessitated frequent and long absences from their posts. The target system gave them little incentive to care about the quality of their work, except for submitting statistical reports indicating that activities were continuing at the targeted level. The more committed health workers in the rural facilities were often frustrated in their attempts to provide better services, since they received little support and no reward for their extra efforts. One hard working health assistant who wanted to improve services at his health post tried to obtain supplies from the district and center. He was unable to see the project chief in Kathmandu or to obtain any supplies. His inspector, while admitting that he was the best health assistant in the district, referred to him in terms implying that he was a troublemaker. If all assistants took such initiatives, he said, there would not be enough money in the district budget to cover even regular activities.

Horizontal Barriers

There were further gaps in the government communication system, not only from the bottom up but also between departments. Because of structural and personality problems, many closely related departments and institutions did not communicate effectively. At the time of my research, the Department of Health Services had little official communication with the Institute of Medicine (IOM), which trained all the health workers for the department's programs. Job descriptions, when they existed, were prepared by the department and not in collaboration with IOM. Nor was there consultation on training curricula. Donor agencies usually avoided working with IOM and the Health Department simultaneously, because even as outsiders they were unable to bridge the internal rivalries. Whatever the reasons for the intensity of this division—and various observers named various causes—it also stemmed from the structure of the central administration, since IOM was responsible to the Ministry of Education and ICHP to the Ministry of Health.

Similarly, in addition to personal rivalries, the historical development of ICHP and its structural position within the Ministry of Health impeded communication and cooperation between ICHP and the vertical projects that were to be integrated. For example, the ICHP chief explained how competition, intensified by the target system, had hindered cooperation between the family planning program and ICHP. Both programs had yearly targets of the number of sterilizations to be done. Since ICHP did not have its own cadre of doctors trained in performing laparoscopies or vasectomies, it had to use doctors from the general service or borrow them from family planning. If a doctor from family planning worked in an ICHP sterilization camp, however, the sterilizations were counted toward the family planning target. Thus, ICHP was reluctant to use family planning doctors because the resulting statistics would favor family planning and undermine ICHP.

The politics of integration have created hostility, resistance, and criticism of an approach to providing health services that in theory most agree has merit. However, the Nepali experience has demonstrated that it is not possible to make successful changes at the local periphery without first making structural changes at the center and providing strong political and administrative support.

Reliance on Quantitative Data

Among the barriers to obtaining accurate information for health planning in Nepal were the difficulty of travel, the limited sources of reliable information, limited access to the decision making process (especially by low-level workers), and the limitation posed by the preference of the decision makers for statistical data. What information was used, and how, depended on the standardized requirements of the donor agencies. In a self-perpetuating exercise, guidelines were formulated at the top of the agency hierarchy and passed down to the field, where data were gathered and reports produced to satisfy the needs of this system.

Economists and administrators in international health agencies typically favor "hard" data, by which they mean statistics that can be used to support cost-benefit analyses and similar economic measurements of a program's financial soundness. Thus, the need to monitor large expenditures and investments determines the kind of information obtained, and "hard" data predominate over "soft" data, such as social and cultural information.

Both the government and donor agencies need quantifiable information to justify creating and securing jobs in the bureaucracy. Government data collection and reports emphasize the quantity, not the quality, of service being provided in order to ensure the continuation of their programs. Problems in the actual delivery of ICHP services thus remained unacknowledged. Since workers at all levels, especially in junior positions, felt unable to solve problems within the program, they directed their efforts instead toward satisfying official requirements.

Donor agencies state that the ultimate objective of financial and technical assistance is to improve health status. Therefore, they emphasize the collection of baseline quantifiable data from which to measure progress—for example, by showing a decrease in infant mortality rates. Often, however, numbers themselves become the goal, as did the targets set in Nepal, and planners lose touch with actual conditions. Trying to improve the quality of life is an indisputably admirable goal, but one that is not easily measurable.

6

Sociocultural Information and the Health Planning Process

In recent years an ever-expanding body of documents from WHO, UNICEF, USAID, and other organizations concerned with international health has stressed the need to utilize in the planning process appropriate sociocultural information obtained through research at the grass roots. Yet there is little evidence that this advice has had much effect. Decisions continue to be made, as in the past, in accordance with a very different system of dynamics—that of successful bureaucracies. And in part the problem lies in the lack of adequate sociocultural information and in a lack of understanding of the research methods that could provide it. And in part the problem stems from certain structural imperatives of all administrative organizations which may prevent relevant information from being used, even when it is available, or in fact, even when it is common knowledge to planners and administrators.

The Anthropologist's Role in Planning

My goal in undertaking this research was to find better ways for health planners and social scientists to

work together. In the course of my work I found that preconceived impressions often intensified misunderstanding.
For example, it is commonly thought that anthropologists
are interested in studying only traditional medical practices
and practitioners. But many anthropologists share with planners an interest in providing effective health care within a
given cultural milieu and in solving the problems faced by
rural health workers. Planners frequently interpret anthropological reports as providing a negative perspective on local
conditions. From the anthropologist's point of view, such information, even if its implications might seem negative, is
directed toward a constructive result.

The planners and administrators I interviewed in Nepal
and in the headquarters of donor agencies often described
social and cultural information as "soft" data, saying that it
was too descriptive, too wordy and confusing, and too difficult to evaluate. They considered anthropologists' reports
to be full of jargon, unwieldy, and unusable; anthropological
studies were described as being "written for the university"
and too narrow in scope. Many planners stated that when
designing a new program, they could not be concerned with
the detailed information on which they feel anthropologists
focus. Since meeting deadlines is very important in the donor agencies, planners tend to see the gathering of anthropological data as too time-consuming, and reports that are
longer than a few pages are resisted. Some agency administrators said that length was not the issue because they simply did not have time to read any background information.
Foreigners did not claim to be familiar with anthropological
information about Nepal. Some Nepali planners and administrators said that they were knowledgeable about rural Nepal's culture, but they agreed with advisors that such
information is often irrelevant to health planning at the central level. Faced with the task of formulating a plan for all
of rural Nepal, planners do not focus on the complexities of
sociocultural information specific to each local area and
group. To take this detailed information into account would
make their task much more complicated. Thus, they tend to
disregard information that is potentially confusing.

Planners' questions about my research also revealed certain preconceived notions about what anthropologists do. One advisor repeatedly asked me why I was studying planners and the planning process instead of studying kinship, as other anthropologists did. This advisor called me his "eyes and ears" because I had more contact than he did with other advisors and with Nepali officials working with ICHP. Ironically, knowledge of Nepali kinship networks could have increased advisors' understanding of decision making within the government. In addition to joking questions about why I did not carry a big stick as Margaret Mead did, I was most frequently asked what "my group" was. When I replied, "the Department of Health," or "health planners," the conversation usually stopped, since this answer definitely did not meet the expectation that anthropologists study a particular ethnic or caste group or village.

This reaction is not surprising. Most of the considerable anthropological literature available on Nepal does focus narrowly on a particular caste or ethnic group. Numerous books, monographs, and dissertations have been written on Brahmans, Chetris, Newars, Gurungs, Magars, Limbus, Sherpas, and Thakalis.[1] Planners do not find this narrow ethnic-caste approach useful. Some planners were aware that a few studies describe interactions among social groups in a particular village or region (Caplan, L. 1970 and 1975; Caplan, P. 1972), and that several excellent historical (Stiller 1973 and 1976) and economic (Regmi 1962, 1976, and 1978) studies describe the political and social integration of Nepal as a unified system. But as they rightly observed, few of these studies attempt to generalize, to focus on the present Nepali social system in national terms, or to look at linkages between the central and local cultures (Rose and Scholz 1980:vii–viii)—in other words, to take a more comprehensive approach that planners would find helpful.

With specific reference to health, several studies were available that planners might have used, including studies of traditional Nepali health beliefs and practices[2] and surveys of health status, some containing information on patients' perceptions of medical services (Worth and Shah 1969; Shah 1978, 1979, 1980, and 1981; Post 1979). Only infrequently did planners mention any of these, although they did cite with interest a journal issue entitled *Anthropology, Health, and Development*[3] that UNICEF was distributing to several donor agencies and government offices at the time of my preliminary research in 1977. Unfortunately, in spite of this show of interest, available health studies appear to have had little effect on planners.

The use of anthropologists by USAID and the World Bank, especially on a contract basis, appears to be increasing, but this trend is less marked in WHO and UNICEF, where few administrators have much confidence in the ability of anthropologists to contribute to achieving program goals. All too often social scientists are hired to fulfill policy mandates and not because senior officials have a real commitment to them or to their potential contributions. The anthropologists who work in the health bureaucracies are frequently criticized for being naive about how planning and administration function. Several agency personnel told me that anthropologists do not understand bureaucracies and lack the planning or administrative experience necessary for working in them. On the other hand, agencies do not know how to use anthropologists effectively. For example, I observed that when agencies did hire social scientists, they often chose people whose training and experience were inappropriate. Social scientists were frequently hired who had no experience or knowledge of Third World countries or of health development. Because agencies rarely have qualified social scientists on their full-time staff, the recommendations made by short-term consulting anthropologists are often taken out of context and adapted to the needs of the system. The view that social scientists have little to offer in the health planning process is thus perpetuated.

Because their role remains in question, anthropologists usually are on the periphery of the planning process. In Nepal, I found few cases where the information they had provided in reports or in "social soundness analyses" had been used. Planners and administrators did not seem to know what to do with cultural and social information when it was available, even though it had been requested by their agencies. When a donor agency funded local social scientists to evaluate survey questionnaires used in Nepal, the lengthy report that resulted was described as being "too philosophical" by administrators, who wanted concrete practical recommendations. And, it must be confessed, the report's frequent use of scholastic terms such as "epistemological" and "ontological" does seem inappropriate, given its audience and purpose. Not surprisingly, this report served to reinforce some of the planners' negative perceptions.

When I interviewed planners, they rarely mentioned needing information from the village level. Any information they did ask for was usually of a statistical nature. For example, when I was preparing to visit District I, a planner asked if I could gather information on methods used by village health workers and at the health post to record causes of death.

International planners frequently mentioned that they wanted more information about the culture of the Nepali government and administration to help agencies improve their relationships with the government. Since the management of health programs in Third World countries had been identified by the agencies as one area needing financial support and technical assistance, some interest was expressed in culture and management—in understanding traditional forms of decision making and how the government works. Thus, when Health Associates, the consulting group contracted by USAID for ICHP, held a half-day seminar in Kathmandu for their consultants in February 1979, two anthropologists were invited to discuss culture and management, to share bibliographic references they had collected, and to propose ways of exploring this area further.

Many foreign planners and consultants come to Nepal with the conviction that their approach to solving health problems is the right one—that they have the answers and do not need to ask questions. They explain their interest in understanding Nepali administration simply as a desire to be able to identify decision makers and to understand the decision making process in order to ensure the acceptance and implementation of their programs. From their point of view, a study of the Nepal government and its administrative processes is the single most important contribution anthropologists might make.

The criticisms of the roles anthropologists and social scientists have played thus far in the health planning process have some validity and help to explain why anthropologists are not taken seriously by health planners. Furthermore, as this study shows, the culture of the planning bureaucracies presents other barriers to using social and cultural information. Yet the disappointing results of programs developed to meet basic health needs continue to suggest that sociocultural factors are relevant to their success.

In considering how anthropologists can help planners de sign more appropriate programs, I reviewed the course of my own research and concluded that in many instances it had not been difficult to understand the cultural appropriateness of the Integrated Community Health Program. Once in the field any sensible observer would see, for example, that VHWs could not visit thirty houses a day and that peons were providing essential health services at rural posts. Understanding how VHWs and peons were viewed by villagers required sensitivity but not extensive anthropological expertise. What anthropologists do have to offer to the planning process is a different approach to gathering information. As an anthropologist, my approach was to visit the rural health facilities, to observe and interview in order to obtain intimate knowledge of the field, and to try to see the program from the Nepali perspective. In contrast, most planners are confined to their offices by the demands of their job and may be less practiced in setting aside their own cultural assumptions. Thus in addition to sociocultural information, the anthropologist's contribution to health planning should include sharing an approach to understanding other cultures.

The following case study of Nepal's Assistant Nurse-Midwife Program demonstrates how I gathered information and used it to evaluate the cultural appropriateness of the ANM's role. This example shows how cultural information commonly known by both Nepalis and foreigners influenced the functioning of a health program, and it then discusses how to incorporate field-level observations into planning.

Using Sociocultural Information to Improve Health Planning: A Case Study[4]

Since the 1960s, the United Nations agencies, especially WHO and UNICEF, and bilateral aid agencies, including USAID, have developed and funded training programs for assistant nurse-midwives (ANMs) as part of national maternal and child health programs. This approach was justified on the grounds that in many countries, Nepal among them, women could be more effective than men in providing maternal and child health care and family planning. Increasing education and employment opportunities through the ANM program was also viewed as a way of enhancing women's social status. Initially designed as part of the basic health services approach to providing care in clinics, the ANM's role was later redefined by international donor agencies and many national governments to include promotive and preventive services, a change that adapted it to community-based primary health care.

To stimulate the development of ANM programs and nursing in general at the country level, WHO sponsored intercountry workshops, provided long- and short-term consultants to governments, and provided international fellowships to strengthen nursing administration and education. WHO and UNICEF also have provided supplies and equipment to support nursing education and services, and bilateral aid has been used for fellowships, curriculum development, and constructing training campuses.

Certainly Nepal has a compelling need for maternal and child health services, since infant and maternal mortality rates there are among the highest in Asia, and childhood diseases are its major health problem. Yet in Nepal, as well as in many other parts of the world, the ANM program has not worked as international agencies and governments expected. Often the ANM has not been able to work effectively because traditional expectations about women conflict with her health role as it has been designed.

The ANM program in Nepal offers two years of training

for women who are at least sixteen years old and who have at least an eighth-grade education. Its stated purpose is to deliver maternal and child health services to the rural population. Based at health posts, the ANMs are responsible for providing prenatal care, delivery services, postnatal care, family planning, and limited infant and child care. They are expected to conduct maternal and child health clinics, including immunizations and health education sessions, and to make home visits to pregnant women, families with young children, and couples eligible for family planning. (See Appendix 3 for ANM job description.)

Although as early as 1965 there were sixteen ANMs working in hospitals (World Health Organization 1978:317), it was not until 1973 as part of a pilot project for integration that they were first assigned to rural health posts and outreach clinics and expected to make home visits on a regular basis (Nepal-Berkeley 1975:237). The number of ANMs increased rapidly during the late 1970s. By 1977 it had grown to 404 (World Health Organization 1978:317); by 1980, 1,049 women had received training from the five ANM training campuses of Tansen, Kathmandu, and three Terai cities (Nepal Ministry of Health 1980). By then the ANM was considered a core worker in Nepal's rural health program, and approximately 60 percent of ANMs were assigned to rural health posts (Nepal Ministry of Health 1980).

Although ANMs were supposed to be trained to work in health posts rather than to serve as staff nurses, by the 1970s the curriculum was primarily in curative medicine, which was more appropriate to clinical settings than to preventive and promotive responsibilities in rural communities. Many ANMs, though technically assigned to health posts and paid as if working there, actually work in hospitals. That they prefer this assignment is understandable, since that is where 90 percent of their training takes place. Here, they fill a gap because there is no government funding for the services they provide in hospitals. Although the 1980 Health Manpower survey indicated how many ANMs had been trained and assigned to hospitals, health centers, and health posts, it did not show how many were actually on duty. According to government reports, all ANM positions in health posts are filled on paper; however, official estimates are that only 30 percent of the ANM health post positions actually have ANMs working in them at any one time (Nepal Ministry of Health 1980:30).

Most ANMs never reach the remote areas to which they are assigned, and those who do rarely remain long. Why? The answer is clear: it is socially unacceptable in Nepal for girls and women to travel and live alone, as ANMs are expected to do. Although there are differing social practices, economic opportunities, and degrees of freedom among the various ethnic and religious groups in Nepal, conservative Hindu values dominate the Nepali view of women: their roles are limited primarily to those of wife and mother. Traditionally, women do not work outside the family but contribute labor to the household and to domestic and agricultural production. Since a woman's status is determined by her marriage—and virtually all women marry—parents are anxious to protect the reputation of their daughters until they can make good matches for them.

ANMs typically come from urban areas, since girls in rural areas, with limited opportunities for education, seldom meet the requirement of an eighth-grade education. In Nepal, the literacy rate for females ten years old and above is 3.7 percent, in contrast to 24.7 percent for males. For females in rural areas, the rate is 2.7 percent, compared to 26.4 percent for those in urban centers (Acharya 1979:28). Although rural educational facilities are increasing, village parents are less willing than urban parents to send girls to school, and rural girls who do go are sent for a shorter time. Some urban families have a more liberal attitude than rural families toward the employment of women outside the home. But though they may view ANM training as an avenue to salaried work, and perhaps to a better marriage, they are in fact often quite unaware of the working situation for which their daughters are being prepared.

Many of the rural health posts to which ANMs are assigned are located in isolated villages, several days' walk from the nearest district center or motorable road. Far from home and family, ANMs must live on their own. If any accommodation is provided at the health post, it usually is occupied by the health assistant, forcing ANMs to find housing in the community. In addition, ANMs are usually the only women working at the post, which makes them especially vulnerable to local criticism and abuse. It is against all sociocultural values for a young, unmarried woman to live on her own in a village or with male staff in a health post. Male workers in rural health posts are often discontented because of the working conditions, especially the isolation from urban areas, but they are not vulnerable in the same sense as women, nor are their reputations at stake.

The social difficulties the ANMs faced were easy to see at the twenty-four health posts I visited. For example, when I arrived at a post in the Terai, in a culturally conservative district of strong Muslim influence which borders on India, I found two ANMs, seventeen and eighteen years old, standing alone at some distance from the male health workers. They gave the impression of being unsure of their role and afraid. Both were from Kathmandu. They were very unhappy at the post and described their situation as difficult. Initially they had had no place to live and had not been accepted by the villagers. They described ways in which the male health workers and villagers had tried to take advantage of them. For example, the senior health assistant expected them to serve both as his assistants in the health post and as personal maids. The girls were also fearful of sexual advances. Although they felt fortunate in having each other for support and in being able to share a rented room in a nearby house, it was difficult for them to adjust to living without water, electricity, and other amenities available in urban areas.

In Nepal's hierarchical society, the urban ANMs were regarded by rural villagers as alien and socially superior. Villagers described their white-and-blue nursing uniforms as "fancy saris" and made remarks about their city shoes. Acceptance in the community is influenced not only by urban-rural differences but also by differing regional attitudes, language barriers, and ethnic and caste distinctions. All outsiders are viewed as strangers, especially when they have different caste and ethnic backgrounds. Reluctant to call upon strangers for help, the villagers continued to rely on family members for pregnancy care, resorting to the health post only when serious problems arose. But even local girls only sixteen years old would be inappropriate as ANMs, because unmarried women without children are viewed as too young and inexperienced to inspire confidence as midwives.

A district doctor who was sensitive to the problems the ANMs were having said that all those in his district were from urban areas and had had great difficulty in adjusting to rural life. He recognized their vulnerability and the obstacles they faced in living and working alone. Those who stayed for a year usually adjusted, he observed, but the only ones who stayed that long were those who could not afford to go home. He cited the lack of field training as another cause of the ANMs' problems.

A nursing consultant also observed that ANMs lack field training. At the ANM campuses, she said, they were treated as though they were in a convent, which fitted with cultural expectations. They then were sent out to work, completely on their own, in total contrast to all cultural expectations. Furthermore, the consultant stated, ANMs were not trained to work independently or to organize and manage their own work, though their job description clearly required these skills.

In the 1979 midterm review of Nepal's health services, health posts reported few prenatal or postnatal clinic activities, family planning services, or home visits (Nepal Ministry of Health 1979). Although primary health care programs stress the ANM's outreach role in the community, there is little incentive for ANMs to leave the safer environment of the post to visit villages. Since they are at the bottom of the health staff hierarchy, ANMs rarely have access to transportation, even when it is available to others at the post.

ANMs are supposed to be supervised by the district public health nurse (PHN), but in 1979 only eight of Nepal's seventy-five districts had PHNs. One PHN told me that she had visited each of the eleven health posts in her district only once during her two-year assignment. In another district, where many health posts are accessible by road, the PHN said she was unable to visit the ANMs because she had no means of transportation and was afraid of being robbed. This PHN was very unhappy in her job. She hoped to be transferred to the capital, where she might obtain a WHO fellowship for further training abroad, which would qualify her for an administrative position in the central Ministry of Health. It was not possible, she said, to lobby for training or promotion from the district. The district doctor, her supervisor, confirmed that she spent most of her time sitting in the district health office complaining and arranging for a transfer back to Kathmandu, and that she was rarely involved in maternal and child health services, even in the district clinics.

Like the ANMs, most PHNs have difficulty adjusting to rural conditions, even in district centers, where adequate accommodations are provided in district hospitals. Even though PHNs usually are older than ANMs and married, and therefore have higher status and greater social acceptance, it is extremely difficult for them to travel on foot or by road to health posts without suitable transport, porter services, and protection. The result is that ANMs receive little support or supervision. Those who do go to rural areas have no choice but to rely on their own limited resources or to give up their jobs and return home, which is a frequent event.

In addition to the social problems faced by the ANMs, their job description often contradicts local customs in relation to pregnancy and child care. As part of WHO's program to upgrade the skills of traditional birth attendants (TBAs), ANMs are instructed to teach pre- and postnatal care and safe methods of delivery to local birth attendants. But in many regions of Nepal, there are no *sudenis* or *dhais* (TBAs). Only 10 percent of rural women receive any kind of formal health care during pregnancy (American Public Health Association 1980:62). Except in the case of complicated deliveries, for which ANMs receive no training, neither ANMs nor TBAs are typically called upon by village women, who rely on themselves and family members for delivery and postnatal care (Parker 1979). In the few areas where there are TBAs, they are mostly older women. It is unlikely that they would welcome suggestions from young unmarried ANMs. Consequently, assigning ANMs to teach TBAs has limited relevance or acceptance in most of Nepal. In 1978 the Institute of Medicine appointed a task force to review the ANM program. Although the task force did not tackle the fundamental problem—that because of social and cultural conditions, the program is inappropriate—some of the basic problems are listed in its report: women are unwilling to go to rural areas; ANMs receive no supervision; and women and children are not being served in the rural areas. The report suggests a solution: existing ANMs should be offered upgraded training to enable them to work in hospitals, while the present rural program should be replaced by a new health auxiliary program that would recruit women from the same areas where they would ultimately work. The curriculum should be redesigned and a pilot training program carried out. However, these sensible recommendations have never been implemented.[5]

Even though in 1979 the Ministry of Health knew that the ANM program was not working, it permitted the Institute of Medicine to proceed with plans to expand the program and open new ANM training campuses. Discussion of expanding the ANM's role in primary health care continued in Kathmandu, just as though the ANMs were functioning satisfactorily.

It is not only planners in Nepal who push ahead despite insurmountable obstacles. When I visited WHO Headquarters in Geneva in June 1979, doctors and planners asked how primary health care was working in Nepal. I discussed the problems of the ANM program with them. Most indicated that they knew of similar problems from personal experience in South Asia and in their own countries. Even in countries with indigenous traditional birth attendants, as young unmarried women ANMs usually find it difficult to gain respect for themselves and their services. One planner was revising policy guidelines for ANM training. But I felt that our discussion was unlikely to influence these guidelines significantly, because the unwelcome evidence, if fully considered, would threaten the very existence of the program.

The low-level peon, the "invisible" worker, is the most accessible health care provider in Nepal's rural health service, despite the fact that his contribution is overlooked by both national and international planners. Ironically, the ANM, her role designed and emphasized by national and international planners, is ineffective, the social and cultural barriers to her success having also been overlooked. Everyone knows that it is socially unacceptable for young unmarried women to live and travel alone in remote villages in Nepal. Several international and government reports recognize that the ANM program does not produce useful health workers for the rural areas.[6] Yet these observations and recommendations are not reflected in the plans and proposals. Thus, the availability of social and cultural information is no guarantee that it will be used.

If the ANM program was in many ways ineffective and culturally antithetical, why was it organized and subsequently continued? One set of answers is political and economic. The program was part of the WHO/UNICEF support package in response to the Nepal government's request for assistance, and accepting it conferred a variety of benefits. Especially after 1975, the International Women's Year, international, national, and private groups were applying pressure for increased employment of women in Nepal. Except for nurses and a few women doctors, most positions in the Nepali health service are filled by men. In the rural health program, men are hired to be family planning motivators, VHWs, and health assistants. The ANM program therefore gave the government an opportunity to show that it was also developing careers for women. Moreover, the foreign assistance available for establishing ANM training schools provided a flow of funds that was difficult to refuse.

To these reasons must be added others that reflect aspects of the bureaucratic cultures described in this study. One aspect is the momentum of international health policy, which inundates local realities as it sweeps downward from policy-making circles to planners in Kathmandu. In a sense, the prevailing health policy is part of the bureaucratic culture of the international donor agencies. Another aspect is the insulation of policymakers and planners from the outcomes of their programs. Since neither Nepali nor foreign planners are involved in implementation, they are shielded from daily reminders of local realities. Still another aspect is the value system of the Western health bureaucracies, which filters out "soft" social and cultural information from the planning and evaluation processes.

A final aspect is the reward systems within the health bureaucracies. Although Nepali civil servants at the Central Secretariat level are aware that many of the plans promoted by the donor agencies are unworkable, they can expect no rewards from either the government or the agencies for voicing their reservations. If they at least appear to cooperate, they can expect rewards in the form of job security and, sometimes, overseas posts with the donor agencies or travel to international conferences. At the same time, they may find ways to obstruct programs they do not believe in or ways to redefine them to fit personal or bureaucratic priorities (Rose and Landau 1977; Scholz and Rose 1980). Foreign planners and consultants, for their part, see themselves as being responsible to offices in Geneva and Washington. Although they may be aware that programs need to be changed, they do not want to make mistakes or take actions that might jeopardize their positions in Nepal or their prospects for advancement. Often they are specialists who are assigned certain tasks over a relatively short term. Their reward lies in successful completion of these tasks, not in criticizing entire programs.

Some Suggestions for Changing the ANM's Role

If the ANM program has not proved effective in providing maternal and child health services in rural areas, it is nevertheless making a variety of positive contributions, both manifest and latent, to hospital care, to the development of nursing cadres, to the expansion of training institutions, to female employment and government manpower lists, to improving individual social status, to increasing purchasing power, and to international agencies, including the provision of jobs for international advisors. A complete dismantling of the program is therefore unlikely, in view of the benefits it brings to the individual, society, government, and international agencies. A more attractive alternative than dismantling is to change the program so that it will be more appropriate to local conditions and needs. Some steps have already been taken in this direction. Nepali health officials have dealt informally with the ANMs' problems by permitting many ANMs to work in hospitals, even though their names remain on the roster of the health post where they are officially assigned and paid. While this solution makes use of the skills ANMs have acquired, it unfortunately bypasses the larger problem of meeting the critical need for maternal and child health services in rural Nepal.

The recruitment of older, married women from the rural areas where they will be posted certainly would be a culturally appropriate alternative to the current practice of hiring young, unmarried urban women. ANMs could then live at home and be available at local health posts and to the nearby community, even though it would still be difficult for them to travel to more distant areas alone. Communities would feel responsible for their own women and would help ensure their protection. Arranging for women to be posted together, even when living with their families, would provide additional support.

Unfortunately, employing older rural women would require lowering the educational requirements for ANM candidates—a change that health officials would be unlikely to make, given the current trend to upgrade and professionalize all health workers. Therefore, I believe that adjusting the existing ANM program to improve its cultural appropriateness gradually is a more realistic strategy. A first step would be to include in the ANM training program an extensive field placement in a rural area for both faculty and students, allowing them to become familiar with local conditions and customs. At one ANM training campus I visited, each student group had a four-week field placement in a village. A foreign nurse, who worked with the government as an ANM tutor, lived with the students in this village, where they met with local leaders, talked with women about local practices for delivery, learned about birth and infancy taboos and rituals, and provided supervised maternal and child health services at the local health post and in mobile clinics in surrounding villages. This was the only such program I observed, but it appeared to be an excellent example of how field experience could be incorporated into the training program. It also illustrated the importance of experience in rural areas for health educators and trainers themselves. Unfortunately, long-term village residence is in some ways easier for a single foreign woman than for her Nepali counterpart. Most female Nepali doctors, nurses, and educators are married women whose husbands work in urban centers; when they go to rural areas, they encounter the same cultural expectations and conflicts as do the ANMs.

Another strategy would be to study traditional birth practices, which vary among ethnic groups and regions, and the role of local women who are called upon to assist in delivery, including older family members and traditional birth attendants. ANMs could incorporate appropriate information learned from these women into their own work with patients.

The few ANMs who have been able to work effectively in rural health posts should be studied to learn what factors have contributed to their success. This information would be useful for determining recruitment criteria as well as for revising training programs. Finally, simplifying the ANMs' job description to limit their responsibilities to those tasks that are most essential and that can be competently done with the available resources would increase their confidence and self-esteem.

In the case of the ANM program, the availability of sociocultural information failed to prevent a culturally inappropriate design from being implemented and maintained; nevertheless, such information may still contribute to making the program more effective. Although sociocultural information cannot ensure culturally appropriate programs, it remains an essential ingredient. Thus anthropologists may make a direct contribution to health planning by sharing their approach, which is to study a situation from the perspective of the participants, thereby providing a missing link between planning and implementation.

Overcoming Obstacles in the Health Bureaucracy

In the world of international health, the choices open to donor agencies are often limited by their own bureaucracies—by their organizational structures, by their planning and funding procedures (which must adhere to certain formats and schedules), and by the organizational and personal goals that influence the planning and evaluation of programs such as ICHP. The demands of the administrative structure and culture often lead donor agencies to a course of action that has more to do with their own needs than with the needs of their beneficiaries.

Although Western administrators and planners may revere rational decision making—choosing the best possible means to an end—planners design programs that conform to their own perceptions, values, and political priorities. Any number of observers have pointed out this phenomenon (see, for example, Goodenough 1976, Rein 1976, and Dror 1971). International planners often attribute failures to the fact that cultural influences can lead people to reject programs. This is undoubtedly true. But the bureaucrats have their own culture, too—one that may obstruct their view of other cultures, resulting in programs that are destined to fail. For example, certain behavior by the donor agencies reflects the need to legitimize decision making. This need leads to a reliance on statistics because they are accepted as validating devices (Devons 1954; Colson 1973). It also leads to the phenomenon of conformity. Different international agencies adopt the same few programs, because failing along with others is less onerous than failing alone. An agency in search of a program is significantly influenced by the course charted by its competitors.

One central problem in providing the best possible health care to rural Nepal is the communication gaps between the cultures involved. The information path between international health policy and its outcomes crosses two major cultural boundaries: one separates the Western "rational" bureaucratic culture of the donor agencies from the Western-ized bureaucratic culture of the Nepal government, with its traditional roots; and the other separates the Nepal govern-ment from the traditional village cultures. Across each boundary information is filtered by the cultural and political environment, and outcomes are accordingly altered. Thus, the concept of integration means one thing to the interna-tional policymakers, something slightly different to the plan-ners in Kathmandu, and still another thing to rural health workers. At each level, efforts are attuned to different goals. And, as the case of ICHP shows, the path for information directed upward from the village level to the health bureau-cracies is even more obstructed than the downward path. Villagers and rural health workers have almost no voice in the planning process. Even when they do speak out, their opinions are usually discounted.

The information used in health planning represents the values of the foreign planners rather than the culture of the local recipients. In practice, the client of the donor agencies is actually the Nepali bureaucracy, not the villagers at whom programs are directed. But the Nepali planners and admin-istrators are also culturally distant from the rural villagers. They, too, function within their own bureaucratic culture. For information from below, they must rely on intermediaries from elite groups who are more skilled at getting medical treatment and other services for themselves. The "poorest of the poor" remain unrepresented.

Despite the primary health care rhetoric about community participation and appropriate health technology, the sophis-ticated administrative, technical, and training requirements to implement the programs sponsored by foreign agencies are beyond present Nepali resources. This means that Nepal must continue to rely upon foreign aid, both financial and technical, and so it continues to be subject to the shifting policies of international planners. The planners may exhaust their interest at the level of planning; Nepali officials must spend their time and energy dealing with representatives of foreign agencies to fulfill the requirements for continued help, at the expense of their own national programs. Con-sequently, for lack of manpower, the provision of health services outside the capital goes largely by default into the hands of those at the bottom. Rural health workers are not linked horizontally in any functioning network, nor are they linked vertically to supportive persons with access to medical supplies, training, or skills. Thus, in spite of all the plans and programs, villagers still have trouble obtaining basic resources for health care.

Despite the considerable obstacles, can social and cultural information improve health planning? The answer will depend not only on efforts by anthropologists and planners to work more closely together but also on changes within the health bureaucracies. During my stay in Nepal, I did detect some hopeful signs.

1. Some outstanding local leaders (e.g., Chittre's district *panchayat* member) find ways to convey local needs and priorities to higher echelons.

2. Voluntary donor agencies, which are usually smaller and less structured than large donor agencies, are often more attuned to local cultures and needs. Often they are able to design programs that are more sensitive to rural priorities (for example, the distribution of drugs by Britain Nepal Medical Trust). These small agencies should be encouraged, and perhaps emulated, to the extent possible.

3. Nepali and foreign planners and administrators were cooperative and generally receptive to the questions raised by this anthropological research. Planners do recognize that some of the problems in delivering health services at present may be related to social and cultural factors and that it is more realistic to change plans than to expect the social and cultural factors to disappear.

4. Donor agencies such as USAID have recently begun encouraging their advisors and representatives to study the Nepali language and to participate in a cultural orientation conducted by a local research group. Foreign consultants stay in villages near health posts. This practice, in conjunction with intensive language study, is a promising way of introducing and sensitizing foreigners to cultural situations.

5. Donor organizations and planners are beginning to rec-

ognize the need for social information, as reflected in their policy statements and requirements for social analysis, even though they are not yet incorporating social and cultural information in their planning.

How can anthropologists and planners work together more fruitfully to gather pertinent sociocultural information and incorporate it into planning and programs? If anthropologists tend to write for themselves and their fellow academics, it can also be said that planners tend to plan for themselves and their fellow planners. Each group needs to understand the other's point of view. Anthropologists need to understand the conditions under which planning is done and the limited alternatives available to planners trying to adopt policies and programs to local cultures. They need to present their information in a form that planners can use. For their part, planners need to understand that sociocultural information is vital and worth the time and money invested in examining it.

In spite of some hopeful signs, there is no easy answer to give anthropologists who want to know how to help improve planning. As long as the structure and culture of health bureaucracies remain unchanged, social and cultural information about people at the grass roots level will have little impact. In designing culturally appropriate programs, the key question is not what information to provide or how to provide it, since the availability of information does not determine its utilization. The key question is how the health bureaucracies can transcend their own cultures to become more sensitive to the cultures they serve.

APPENDIXES

APPENDIX 1

A Chronology of Health-Sector Events in Nepal

Year	Popu-lation × 10⁶	Physi-cians	Other health workers: Training	Planning	Services development		
					Categorical programs	Hospitals	Health posts
1925	5.5				Malaria survey		
1934		1	Civil Medical School (CMS)				
1952	8.7	12	WHO, USAID Participant training			33	0
1954				Rapti Valley (Chitwan) Multi-Sector Development			
1956			Health Assistant Training School (HATS).	1st Plan: Hospitals upgraded; Ministry of Health organized	Malaria pilot project 2,000,000 cases		24
1958			NMEO begins to train 100s of workers		NMEO formed		

1962	9.8		450 auxiliaries since 1934	2d Plan: Hospitals upgraded; manpower planning	Smallpox		
1964					MCH		9
1965				National Health Survey	TB/Leprosy; FP/MCH	36	
1971	11.4	311	900 nurses and auxiliaries		UNICEF Community Water Supply Project		153
1972			Ministry of Education/Institute of Medicine takes over training most auxiliaries	Kaski-Bara Pilot; Integrated Health System	2,500 cases of malaria		
1974		288		Planning cell in MOH	Last case of smallpox; malaria resurges	58	251
1975	12.9	348	Over 1,000 health workers trained by IOM; DHS trains VHWs; FP/MCH trains panchayat-based workers (PBWs)	5th Plan: Formulation for nationwide integrated health services; National Nutrition Survey	FP/MCH expands to all districts; malaria program revitalized		351

					Services development		
Year	Population × 10⁶	Physi-cians	Other health workers: Training	Planning	Categorical programs	Hospitals	Health posts
1978	13.9	375	About 1,000 VHW, 450 FP/PBWs, 2,000 health-post and hospital midlevel workers; over 3,000 malaria workers	*Presumptive Sixth Plan:* Push for integration of all rural health services	Malaria stable; smallpox program turns to other immunizations; increase in sterilizations; expanded primary care	69	483 (233 integrated)
1979	14.0 (est.)	457	About 270 VHWs, 77 ANMs, 34 AHWs, 61 HPIs* and 500 PBHWs provided in-service training; 10 ob/gyns provided laprocator-minilap training; 25 physicians trained in vasectomy	*Sixth Plan:* Revised to postpone development of ward-level health workers	48 district health offices in operation; 13 fully integrated districts; increase in sterilization services provided at mobile camp and permanent centers; malaria field tests malathion	70	533 (283 integrated)

Note: Dates given in chart may indicate when activities began and not the official inauguration of a program.
*HPI—Health worker in-charge of Health Post.

SOURCE: Health Associates 1978

APPENDIX 2

Profile of Health Workers in ICHP

Health worker	Educational requirement	Where educated	Source	Responsibilities
Village Health Worker (VHW)	8th Grade plus in-service training.	ICHP in-service training of one month.	Vertical projects; local recruitment by chief district officer.	Regular home visits to all families in defined area for family planning motivation and services, communicable disease and nutritional surveillance and oral rehydration.
Auxiliary Health Worker (AHW)	8th or 10th grade plus AHW course or vertical-project supervisory experience.	IOM, Lazimpat, and Birgunj campuses; 1-year (10th grade) or 2-year (8th grade) course.	IOM graduates; vertical projects.	Assist HA in curative and preventive services at health post and in supervision of VHW.
Assistant Nurse-Midwife (ANM)	8th grade plus ANM course.	IOM, several campuses; 1½-year course.	IOM graduates.	Manage FP/MCH activities at health post and outreach clinics, provide midwifery services in health post area, and supervise VHW in FP/MCH activities.

Senior Auxiliary Health Worker (SAHW)	AHW or earlier compounder or equivalent course, plus work experience and upgrading course.	IOM upgrading course of several weeks' duration	AHW or equivalent.	Equivalent to HA, acts as HA in health post management and supervision.
Health Assistant (HA)	10th grade plus certificate course.	IOM, Maharajganj Campus; 2½-year course.	IOM graduates.	Manage health post, supervise curative and preventive services provided by health post and fieldworkers.
Health Inspector (HI)	At least 10th grade (some B.A. or higher), plus work experience and in-service training.	ICHP in-service training of 2 to 4 weeks.	Vertical projects, HAs.	Manage district health office (48 sanctioned) and supervise health-post operations.
Medical Officer (MO)	M.B.B.S. or equivalent.	India, other foreign universities.	M.B.B.S. graduates.	Curative services at district hospitals, administrative and technical responsibility for district health offices, surgical family planning services at hospitals and in camps.

SOURCE: Health Associates 1978

APPENDIX 3

Job Descriptions for ICHP
Workers (Unofficial translation from
Nepali text)

Functions of Community Health
Volunteer

1. To remain conscious of the ward's* problems related to health and family planning and also make the people aware of these problems.

2. To carry out activities with the people's participation in order to improve the health of the local people and to protect them from diseases.

3. To assist the people in making maximum use of locally available health facilities (health post, Ayurvedic clinics, drinking water, kitchen garden, etc.).

4. To motivate married couples to use family planning.

5. To distribute pills and condoms to willing married couples.

6. To lend necessary assistance in establishing vasectomy

*Each village *panchayat* is divided into nine wards with approximately equal population.

6. To lend necessary assistance in establishing vasectomy camps according to the demand of the local people by keeping in touch with the health post and public health office.

7. To carry out follow-up work in the case of couples using family planning facilities and refer them to the health post.

8. To motivate the people to immunize children (one to twelve months old) and bring them to the ward vaccination clinic at definite times in the campaign to immunize children as a means of preventing epidemics.

9. To help in the establishment of the ward vaccination clinic and assist in the work.

10. To lend manpower assistance to the health post and rural health workers in preserving vaccines by storing them in cold chain.

11. To collect blood samples to diagnose people with fever.

12. To give presumptive treatment to those fever cases whose slides have been taken.

13. To adopt and help people adopt measures to prevent malaria—keeping the house and surrounding area clean, using mosquito nets, filling ditches and trenches to avoid the accumulation of water, planting saplings, and so on.

14. To refer patients suspected of tuberculosis or leprosy to VHWs and the health post.

15. To remind the confirmed tuberculosis and leprosy cases to take the medicine given to them by the VHW regularly.

16. Each ward-level panchayat health worker should arrange a specific place to conduct health education classes and seminars with the cooperation and active participation of the concerned ward committee and the people. Immunization clinics shall also be based in the same place.

17. To arrange at least two exhibitions every month of health education activities and materials at the ward-level health education center regarding nutrition, personal and environmental sanitation (methods of proper disposal of night soil, urine, dirt and garbage, etc.), family planning/maternal and child health activities, and control and prevention of epidemics.

energy malnutrition condition of children one to five years old and to diagnose and control tuberculosis among children of this age group in the villages.

19. To provide intensive education regarding nutrition.

20. To provide intensive education about the use of "Aushadhi paani" rehydration fluid to protect people from dying of diarrhea.

21. To provide necessary education on safe home-delivery practices and on disinfecting the naval-severing knife and other related matters.

22. To tell the local sudenis (traditional birth attendants) to contact the local integrated health post for necessary training.

23. To help form the Ward Health Committee and work as secretary of that committee.

24. To maintain statistics of births and deaths in the ward and submit its report to the VHW every month.

25. In the event of an outbreak of an epidemic, to report immediately to the health post, district health office, and the hospital.

26. To provide first aid treatment and refer other patients to the health post for appropriate treatment.

27. To make use of specific Ayurvedic herbs for providing first-aid treatment.

Village Health Worker (VHW) Job Description

The VHW is responsible to the Health-Post In-charge through the Auxiliary Health Worker (AHW[P]).

The following are the jobs to be performed by him as daily routine in the field.

I. General Field Activities

    1. Checks his visiting bag to be sure that all the supplies needed, including the correct village health records VHRs, are taken before making the daily round.

    2. Follows the prescribed routine of activities for each house visit.

    3. Records all particulars in the VHR.

    4. Updates the stencil at each house visit.

    5. Visits every house in the Vek once a month and tries to contact as many family members as possible.

II. Enumeration and Updating of Household Information. Finds out whether there have been any births, deaths, marriages or settlers (not visitors) or new houses constructed since his last visit and records the information in the VHR.

III. Malaria

    1. Determines if anyone in the household or any visitor has a fever or has had a fever since his last visit.

    2. Takes blood and prepares slide according to prescribed procedure of anyone who has a fever or has had a fever.

    3. Gives presumptive treatment as prescribed.

    4. Takes blood slides from all positive malaria cases for 12 consecutive months; if there is refusal, reports to AHW(P).

IV. Smallpox

    1. Determines if anyone in the household or any visitor has a rash.

    2. If a rash with illness is detected, examines it.

    3. Reports all rashes with illness immediately to the Health Post.

    4. Vaccinates and revaccinates according to the prescribed schedule on an annual basis.

V. Hansen's Disease

    1. Observes for apparent signs of Hansen's disease during interaction with people in the house and encourages anyone with signs of the disease to visit the Health Post for check-up.

    2. Checks on his non-surveillance (reporting) days whether the referred case has attended the Health Post for check-up; if not, encourages the suspected case again to go to the Health Post.

    3. If a person is diagnosed as having the disease, en-

courages the person to take the prescribed treatment regularly.

4. Visits the diagnosed case every month to check whether the prescribed treatment is being continued; if not, reports to the AHW(P).

5. Reminds the case about when to return to the Health Post for follow-up.

VI. Other Diseases

1. Encourages any person complaining of other illnesses to go to the Health Post for check-up and treatment.

2. Reports any severe case of diarrhea or vomiting with diarrhea to the Health Post In charge.

3. Reports any illness in unusual numbers to the Health Post In-charge.

VII. MCH

1. In the MCH's field area (home visiting area), furnishes names and addresses to the ANM of:
   —sick children, especially those not getting enough food, and diarrhea cases.
   —newborns.
   —pregnant women (to report once during the period of pregnancy).

2. In all areas, finds out sick children
   —if the sickness is due to diarrhea, explains and shows making of special water mixture (salt-sugar-water) and encourages the mothers to give food to the sick children.
   —even if the sickness is not due to diarrhea, encourages the mother to give more food and water frequently.
   —refers the sick children to be taken by the mothers to the Health Post for check-up and treatment.

3. If any child has visible thin ribs, thin legs, arms and pot belly, face like an old person, encourages the mother to give more food and mixed foods frequently; refers the child to be taken by the mother to the Health Post for check-up and treatment.

4. If any child has a puffy pale look, swelling of the legs or entire body, dull to light colored hair, and no energy, encourages the mother to give more food and mixed foods frequently; refers the child to be taken by the mother to the Health Post for check-up and treatment.
5. Encourages all pregnant women to attend the antenatal clinics.
6. Encourages all mothers to have their children immunized and stresses the 12 points for the 'Health of the Child.'

VIII. Family Planning
1. Identifies all the eligible couples and motivates them to use either temporary or permanent contraceptive methods.
2. Refers those couples eligible and willing for permanent contraceptive methods (sterilization) or loop-insertion to the district or zonal hospital.
3. If no contraindications are apparent, explains the exact use of the pill to those couples desiring to use pill and provides the couples with two cycles of pills initially.
4. When contraindications for using the pill are apparent, encourages the women to go to the Health Post for counseling and evaluation.
5. Explains how to use the condom to those men desiring to use condom and provides fifteen condoms initially.
6. Explains to the couple how to get a resupply of either condoms or contraceptive pills.
7. On monthly visits:
   —encourages continuation of the contraceptive method accepted.
   —determines if contraceptives are being used correctly.
   —provides relief for minor side-effects due to the pill and refers those with major side-effects to the Health Post.
   —resupplies couples with needed contraceptives.

—continues motivation for those not yet accepting one of the family planning methods.

IX. Health Education—General

1. Uses both individual and group communication methods during house visits.
2. Attempts to motivate people with regard to improved health behavior by following, whenever possible, the four simple rules of motivation.
3. Establishes good interpersonal relations with people in the community.

Health Education Regarding Specific Activities

1. Provides individuals and families with correct messages concerning each of the health activities.
2. Answers questions about the various health activities with correct information.
3. Works in cooperation with other Health Post staff in solving special health problems.

X. When Working at the Health Post on Non-Surveillance (Reporting) Days

1. Records all the prescribed information of his Vek in the CHRs.
2. Prepares all the required forms and reports as prescribed.
3. Obtains instructions from the Health Post In-charge, AHW(P) and ANM about all referrals made by him to the Health Post and about follow-ups needed pertaining to family planning, positive malaria cases, and newly diagnosed cases of tuberculosis and leprosy.

XI. The female JAHW will assist the ANM with her routine duties.

Assistant Nurse-Midwife (ANM) Job Description

The ANM is responsible to the Health Post In-Charge. She is responsible:

1. for receiving supervision and technical guidance from the Public Health Nurse of the district.
2. for providing antenatal care, delivery service, postnatal care, and infant and child care.
3. for conducting health education sessions on her clinic days; of the various subjects dealt with, nutrition education relating to the feeding of children from 6 months to two years of age, prevention and treatment of diarrhea including rehydration therapy and the 12 Points for the Health of the Child will be stressed. These health education sessions should include appropriate demonstrations of how to do what is being taught.
4. for providing immunization service.
5. for conducting deliveries at the Health Post where adequate facilities exist.
6. for assisting the Health Post In-charge with the provision of curative care on the 'General Activity' day, and on Antenatal Clinic day when time is available.
7. for providing curative care during the absence of both the Health Post In-charge and the AHW(C).
8. for sharing with the Health Post In-charge the care of equipment, sterilization, safe practices in the Health Post, maintaining kits including midwifery kit in readiness, housekeeping, general cleanliness, etc.
9. for providing the JAHWs with technical guidance and advice for MCH/FP activities on the reporting days at the Health Post and on home-visiting days.
10. for assisting the Health Post In-charge with the in-service training of staff, especially in the field of MCH/FP.
11. for keeping all relevant records properly and up-to-date and for submitting the required reports promptly.
12. for visiting the homes of mothers and children identified at the Health Post and Outreach Clinics who require special MCH care.
13. for searching for pregnant women, to encourage them to attend the antenatal clinic and provide antenatal care at the home.
14. for searching for all newborns not attended by her already in order to provide neonatal care and nutrition education and postnatal care for the mothers concerned.

15. for encouraging mothers to bring their children to the Children's Clinics at the Health Post/Outreach Clinic for well baby care, i.e., weighing, immunization, nutrition demonstration, etc. and to update the Road to Health Card.

16. for identifying the total family needs in the homes visited for MCH services and for preparing an MCH care plan for those families that need this service.

17. for conducting home deliveries and making necessary referrals, as required, and for following up the mothers for postnatal care and babies for infant care.

18. for keeping in close contact with the local birth attendants to teach and encourage them to follow safe methods of delivery, antenatal, postnatal, and infant care and in family planning activities.

19. for encouraging eligible couples to accept appropriate contraceptive methods.

20. for visiting pill acceptors in the home-visiting area who have been referred by the JAHW for special follow-up, i.e., side effects, drop-outs, remotivation, etc.; and for following up loop acceptors.

21. for assisting in the organization and conduct of laparoscopy and loop-insertion camps.

22. for assisting as a disease surveillance agent during her clinic sessions and home visits and for reporting to the Health Post In-charge on the occurrence of smallpox, cholera, or other diseases in unusual numbers; and to take blood smears from fever cases for malaria surveillance.

23. for cultivating good relations with the community as a member of the Health Post staff to obtain community cooperation for the efficient discharge of her duties.

Notes

1. Introduction

1. Among cross-cultural studies of bureaucracy appearing recently, Cohen's (1980) analysis of the Nigerian bureaucracy and Rosen's (1980) study of provincial administration in Ethiopia document how bureaucratic forms differ and reflect informal social organization. Conkling's study (1979) of authority and change in Indonesian bureaucracy contrasts Western and Third World bureaucracies. Foster (1969; 1969b; 1976) has discussed the importance of using a holistic anthropological analysis in studying the structure and functioning of bureaucracies as social and cultural systems. Britan and Cohen's (1980) recent collection of articles, a valuable contribution to the anthropological study of bureaucracy, provides a number of instances of the application of comparative analysis and ethnographic method to the study of complex organizations.

2. For more detailed discussion of traditional medicine in Nepal see: Allen 1976; Bennett 1976; Blaustain 1976; Hitchcock 1975; Hitchcock and Jones 1976; Hoffer 1974a, 1974b; Jones 1978; Macdonald 1975; Michl 1974; Miller 1979; Okada

1976; Parker et al. 1979; Stablein 1973, 1976a, 1976b, 1976c, 1976d; Stone 1976; Wake 1976; Watters 1975.

3. External agencies involved in health activities in Nepal in April 1979 were the following: Bilateral agencies— Australian Development Assistance Bureau, Canadian International Development Agency, Federal Republic of Germany, Indian Cooperation Mission, Japanese International Cooperation Agency, Japanese Organization for Volunteers Overseas, Netherlands Government, British Overseas Development Ministry, U.S. Peace Corps, Swiss Association for Technical Assistance, U.S. Agency for International Development, British Voluntary Service Overseas, Union of Soviet Socialist Republics; International Agencies—U.N. Food and Agriculture Organization, International Bank for Reconstruction and Development, International Development Association, U.N. Development Programme, U.N. Fund for Population Activities, U.N. Children's Fund, U.N. World Health Organization; Voluntary—Alberta, Canada (ALTA), Australia Youth Council for Development Assistance, Britain Nepal Medical Trust, Evangelical Mission, Himalayan Trust, International Nepal Fellowship, Japanese Organization for International Cooperation in Family Planning, Leprosy Mission, Netherlands Leprosy Relief Association, Save the Children Fund, Seventh Day Adventist Mission, Sasakawa Memorial Health Foundation, Thomas Dooley Foundation, United Mission to Nepal, Unitarian Society of Canada, World Food Program, World Neighbors.

2. Health Bureaucracies: Structure and Culture

1. For further discussion on administration in Nepal: Agrawal 1976; Goodall 1963; Joshi 1973; Pradhan 1976; Rose and Landau 1978; Rose and Scholz 1979 and 1980; Schloss 1980; Shrestha 1975. References on Nepali politics include Baral 1978; Chauhan 1971; Gupta 1964; Joshi and Rose 1966; Muni 1977; Nath 1975; Rose and Fisher 1970; Shaha 1975b.

2. In comparing how villages in different regions dealt with the central bureaucracy, Scholz (1981:34) found regional differences in involvement with the center's development programs depending on the intermediate linkage system. Where informal networks were more numerous and stronger, local acceptance of central programs was greater.

3. See Chap. 1, n. 3.

4. See Hoben 1980:350 for detailed discussion of this procedure.

3. Policies and Plans

1. USAID, Population Planning and Health Programs, Obligations/Loans Authorizations/Planning Levels Fiscal Years 1965–1981.

2. The program (ICHP) was variously called Community Health and Integration, Integrated Community Health Division, Integrated Community Health Services, Integrated Community Health Project, and Integrated Community Health Services Development Project in different documents and at different times.

3. Insufficient information is one of many reasons given for the failure of planning in Nepal (Wildavsky 1972).

4. In fact, by 1979, administrative and budgetary changes made the Integrated Community Health Program equivalent to a vertical project.

4. Delivering Services to Rural Villages

1. See Parker 1979 for a survey of traditional birth attendants in Nepal.

2. See chap. 1 n. 2 on traditional medicine in Nepal.

3. This section has previously been published in a longer version: "The Invisible Worker: The Role of the Peon in Ne-

pal's Health Service," *Social Science and Medicine* 17(14): 967–970, 1983.

5. Sources and Channels of Information

1. See Hoben 1980:348–350 for a detailed description of USAID's preparation and review of policy and program-budget documents, the central activity for AID's line-organization units, the regional bureaus, and the country missions: "It occupies much of the time of their employees and takes precedence over all other activities."
2. See Chambers 1980 for discussion of "rural development tourism"—the phenomenon of the brief rural visit.

6. Sociocultural Information and the Health Planning Process

1. Anthropological literature available on Nepal's ethnic groups: Bista 1967; Caplan, L. 1970, 1975; Caplan, P. 1972; Furer-Haimendorf 1964, 1966, 1974, 1975; Hitchcock 1966; Jones and Jones 1976; Macfarlane 1976; Messerschmidt 1976; Nepali 1965. The *Himalayan Research Bulletin,* published four times yearly, lists current Ph.D. dissertations on Nepal.
2. See chap. 1 n. 2 on traditional medicine in Nepal.
3. *Contributions to Nepalese Studies* 1976, special issue on "Anthropology, Health and Development."
4. This section has previously been published in a longer version: "Can Sociocultural Information Improve Health Planning? A Case Study of Nepal's Assistant Nurse-Midwife," *Social Science and Medicine* 19(3):193–198, 1984.
5. This discussion describes the ANM training as it was in 1979. Although the curriculum has been changed since then, it is unknown whether this has altered the role of the ANM in rural areas.

6. Recognition of problems in Nepal's Assistant Nurse-Midwife Program is made in the following reports: *Mid-Term Health Review* (Nepal Ministry of Health 1979), *Health Manpower Survey* (Nepal Planning Unit, Ministry of Health 1980), *Assistant Nurse-Midwife Task Force Report* (Mimeo. 1978), *An Evaluation of AID-Financed Health and Family Planning Projects in Nepal* (American Public Health Association 1980).

Bibliography

Acharya, Meena
1979 Statistical Profile of Nepalese Women: A Critical Review. *In*
The Status of Women in Nepal. Volume 1: Background Report,
Part 1. Kathmandu: Centre for Economic Development and
Administration.
Agrawal, Hem Narayan
1976 The Administrative System of Nepal: From Tradition to
Modernity. New Delhi: Vikas.
Allen, N. J.
1976 Approaches to Illness in the Nepalese Hills. *In* Social An-
thropology and Medicine. Joseph B. Loudon, ed. Pp. 500–552.
New York, San Francisco, London: Academic Press.
American Public Health Association
1980 An Evaluation of AID-Financed Health and Family Planning
Project in Nepal. Washington: American Public Health
Association.
Anderson, Mary M.
1971 The Festivals of Nepal. London: George Allen and Unwin
Ltd.
Bainbridge, J., and S. Sapirie
1974 Health Project Management: A Manual of Procedures for
Formulating and Implementing Health Projects. Geneva: World
Health Organization.
Banerji, D.
1973 Health Behavior of Rural Populations: Impact of Rural
Health Services. Economic and Political Weekly (22 December).
Banskota, Mahesh
1983 Foreign Aid and the Poor: Some Observations on Nepal's

Experience. *In* Foreign Aid and Development in Nepal. Proceedings of a Seminar (October 4–5, 1983). Pp. 35–82. Kathmandu: Integrated Development Systems.

Baral, Lok Raj
1978 Oppositional Politics in Nepal. Columbia, Mo.: South Asia Books.

Barth, Frederick
1966 Models of Social Organization. London: Royal Anthropological Institute.

Bennett-Campbell, Lynn
1974 Pregnancy, Birth and Early Child Rearing: Health and Family Planning Attitudes and Practices in a Brahman-Chetri Community. Research-cum Action Project. Paper No. 9. Kathmandu: Department of Local Development/UNICEF.
1976 Sex and Motherhood Among the Brahmans and Chetris of East-Central Nepal. Contributions to Nepalese Studies 3 (Special Issue): 1–52.

Berry, Sara S.
1980 Decision Making and Policy Making in Rural Development. *In* Agricultural Decision Making: Anthropological Contributions to Rural Development. Peggy F. Barlett, ed. Pp. 321–336. New York: Academic Press.

Bhooshan, B. S.
1979 The Development Experience of Nepal. New Delhi: Concept Publishing.

Bista, Dor Bahadur
1967 People of Nepal. Kathmandu: Ratna Pustak Bhandar.

Blaikie, Piers, John Cameron, and David Seddon
1980 Nepal in Crisis: Growth and Stagnation at the Periphery. Delhi: Oxford University Press.

Blum, H. L.
1978 Observations and Recommendations on the Family Planning-Maternal and Child Health Services of the Ministry of Health of Nepal and Their Relationship to the Development of Goals of His Majesty's Government. Berkeley: For Nepal-Berkeley Family Planning/Maternal Child Health Project.

Blustain, Harvey S.
1976 Levels of Medicine in a Central Nepali Village. Contributions to Nepalese Studies 3 (Special Issue): 83–105.

Borgstrom, Bengt-Erik
1976 Thoughts on the Relevance of Social Anthropology for Development Planning: The Case of Nepal. *In* Development from

Below: Anthropologists and Development Situations. David C. Pitt, ed. Pp. 83–95. The Hague: Mouton.

1980 The Patron and the Panca: Village Values and Democracy in Nepal. New Delhi: Vikas Publishing House Pvt. Ltd.

Britan, Gerald M., and Ronald Cohen, eds.

1980 Hierarchy and Society: Anthropological Perspectives on Bureaucracy. Philadelphia: Institute for Study of Human Issues, Inc.

Britton, Margaret

1978 A Proposed Model for Community Participation in Health, Family Planning and Nutrition. Kathmandu: USAID/Nepal.

Brockington, Fraser

1975 World Health. Edinburgh: Churchill Livingston.

Brown, Richard

1976 Public Health as Imperialism: Early Rockefeller Programs at Home and Abroad. American Journal of Public Health 66(9): 897–906.

1979a Exporting Medical Education: Professionalism, Modernization, and Imperialism. School of Public Health, University of California, Los Angeles. Unpublished manuscript.

1979b Rockefeller Medicine Men: Medicine and Capitalism in America. Berkeley, Los Angeles, London: University of California Press.

Bryant, John

1969 Health and the Developing World. Ithaca: Cornell University Press.

Campbell, G., Ramesh Shrestha, and Linda Stone

1979 The Use and Misuse of Social Science Research in Nepal. Kathmandu: Research Center for Nepal and Asian Studies, Tribhuvan University.

Caplan, A. Patricia

1972 Priests and Cobblers: A Study of Social Change in a Hindu Village in Western Nepal. San Francisco: Chandler Publishing Co.

Caplan, Lionel

1970 Land and Social Change in East Nepal: A Study of Hindu-Tribal Relations. London: Routledge and Kegan Paul.

1972 District Administration as an Arena for Local Leadership Struggles: A Nepalese Case. Paper given at Conference on Leadership in South Asia, School of Oriental and African Studies, London, 11 May.

1975 Administration and Politics in a Nepalese Town: The Study of a District Capital and Its Environs. London: Oxford University Press.

Cardinalli, Robert J.
1979 Population-Related Social Research in Nepal. Kathmandu: United Nations Fund for Population Activities.

Chambers, Robert
1979 Rural Health Planning: Why Seasons Matter. IDS Working Paper. Brighton, England: Institute of Development Studies.
1980 Rural Poverty Unperceived: Problems and Remedies. World Bank Staff Working Paper, No. 400. Washington: World Bank.

Chauhan, R. S.
1971 The Political Development in Nepal, 1950–1970. New Delhi: Associated.

Chowdhari, Seeta Ram
1979 Report on Family Planning/Health Delivery System in Nepal. Kathmandu: United Nations Fund for Population Activities.

Clugston, Graeme A.
1978 The Britain Nepal Medical Trust: An Analysis of Present and Future Programs. London: London School of Hygiene and Tropical Medicine.

Cochrane, Glynn
1980 Policy Studies and Anthropology. Current Anthropology 21(4): 445–458.

Cohen, Ronald
1980 The Blessed Job in Nigeria. In Hierarchy and Society: Anthropological Perspectives on Bureaucracy. Gerald M. Britan and Ronald Cohen, eds. Pp. 73–88. Philadelphia: Institute for the Study of Human Issues, Inc.

Colson, Elizabeth
1973 Tranquility for the Decision-Maker. In Culture, Illness and Health: Essays in Human Adaptation. Laura Nader and Thomas W. Maretzki, eds. Washington: American Anthropological Association.
1982 Planned Change: The Creation of a New Community. Berkeley: Institute of International Studies, University of California.

Conkling, Robert
1979 Authority and Change in Indonesian Bureaucracy. American Ethnologist 6(3): 543–554.

Devons, Eli
1954 Statistics as a Basis for Policy. Lloyds Bank Review (n.s) 33: 30–43.

Djukanovic V., and E. P. Mach, eds.
1975 Alternative Approaches to Meeting Basic Health Needs in Developing Countries: A Joint UNICEF/WHO Study. Geneva: World Health Organization.

Dror, Yehezkel
1971 Design for Policy Sciences. New York: American Elsevier Publishing Co., Inc.

Dunn, Frederick L.
1962 Medical-Geographical Observations in Central Nepal. Millbank Memorial Fund Quarterly 15(2): 125–148.
1977 Personal communication.

Eddy, Elizabeth, and William Partridge, eds.
1978 Applied Anthropology in America. New York: Columbia University Press.

Evans, John R., Karen Lashman Hall, and Jeremy Warfend
1981 Shattuck Lecture—Health Care in the Developing World: Problems of Scarcity and Choice. The New England Journal of Medicine 305(19): 1117–1127.

Family Health Care, Inc.
1979 Planning for Health and Development: A Strategic Perspective for Technical Cooperation. Volume I and II. Washington: USAID, Office of Health.

Fletcher, Grace Nies
1964 The Fabulous Flemings of Kathmandu: The Story of Two Doctors in Nepal. New York: E. P. Dutton and Co., Inc.

Foster, George M.
1969a An Anthropologist's View of Technical Assistance Methodology. University of California, Berkeley. Unpublished manuscript.
1969b Applied Anthropology. Boston: Little, Brown and Company.
1976 Medical Anthropology and International Health Planning. Medical Anthropology Newsletter 7(3): 12–18.
1982 Community Development and Primary Health Care: Their Conceptual Similarities. Medical Anthropology 6:183–195.

Furer-Haimendorf, Christoph von
1964 The Sherpas of Nepal: Buddhist Highlanders. Berkeley and Los Angeles: University of California Press.
1966 Caste and Kin in Nepal, India and Ceylon: Anthropological Studies in Hindu-Buddhist Contact Zones. New Delhi: Sterling Publishers Pvt. Ltd.
1974 Contributions to the Anthropology of Nepal. Warminster, England: Aris and Phillips Ltd.

1975 Himalayan Traders: Life in Highland Nepal. London: John Murray.

Gaige, Frederick H.
1975 Regionalism and National Unity in Nepal. Berkeley, Los Angeles, London: University of California Press.

Gautam, Prasanna Chandra
1974 Health Problems in Karnali Zone: A Hospital-based Comprehensive Study. Kathmandu: UNICEF.

Geertz, Clifford
1973 The Interpretation of Culture. New York: Basic Books.

Geilhufe, Nancy L.
1979 Anthropology and Policy Analysis. Current Anthropology 20(3): 557–579.

Goldstein, Melvyn C., and Cynthia M. Beall
1981 Modernization and Aging in the Third and Fourth World: Views from the Rural Hinterland in Nepal. Human Organization 40(1): 48–55.

Golladay, Frederick, and Bernard Liese
1980 Health Problems and Policies in the Developing Countries. World Bank Staff Working Paper, No. 412. Washington, D.C: World Bank.

Goodall, Merrill R.
1963 Development of Public Administration in Nepal. Final Report to the Government of Nepal. Kathmandu: United Nations Technical Assistance Program.
1966 Administrative Change in Nepal. In Asian Bureaucratic Systems Emergent from the British Imperial Tradition. Ralph Braibanti, ed. Pp. 605–642. Durham, N.C.: Duke University Press.

Goodenough, Ward
1976 Intercultural Expertise and Public Policy. In Anthropology and the Public Interest. Peggy Sanday, ed. Pp. 15–24. New York: Academic Press.

Goodman, Neville M.
1971 International Health Organizations and Their Work. Edinburgh: Churchill Livingstone.

Gupta, Anirudha
1964 Politics in Nepal. Bombay: Allied Publishers.

Gurung, Harka
1978 Distribution Pattern and Cost of Administration in Nepal. Journal of Development and Administrative Studies 1(1): 1–18.

Gwatkins, Davidson R., Janet R. Wilcox, and Joe D. Wray
1980 Can Health and Nutrition Interventions Make a Difference? Washington: Overseas Development Council.

Hagen, Toni
1961 Nepal: The Kingdom in the Himalayas. Berne: Kummerly and Frey.
Hall, Douglas E., and Alan E. Dieffenbach
1973 Compensation of Foreign Advisors in Development Countries. IDR/Focus 3:1–6.
Harwood, Alan
1978 Discussion on John Janzen's Paper. Social Science and Medicine 12:131–133.
Health Associates
1979 Personal communication, 13 April.
Heighton, Robert H., and Christy Heighton
1978 Applying the Anthropological Perspective to Social Policy. In Applied Anthropology in America. Elizabeth Eddy and William Partridge, eds. Pp. 390–411. New York: Columbia University Press.
Hitchcock, John T.
1963 Some Effects of Recent Change in Rural Nepal. Human Organization 22:75–83.
1966 The Maggars of Banyan Hill. New York: Holt, Rinehart and Winston.
1974 A Shaman's Song and Some Implications for Himalayan Research. In The Anthropology of Nepal. Christoph von Furer-Haimendorf, ed. Pp. 150–156. Warminster, England: Aris and Phillips.
1976 Spirit Possession in the Nepal Himalayas. New Delhi: Vikas Publishing House.
Hoben, Allan
1980 Agricultural Decision Making in Foreign Assistance: An Anthropological Analysis. In Agricultural Decision Making: Anthropological Contributions to Rural Development. Peggy F. Barlett, ed. Pp. 337–371. New York: Academic Press.
Hofer, Andras
1974a A Note on Possession in South-Asia. In The Anthropology of Nepal. Christoph von Furer-Haimendorf, ed. Pp. 159–167. Warminster, England: Aris and Phillips.
1974b Is the Bombo an Ecstatic? Ritual Techniques of Tamang Shamanism. In The Anthropology of Nepal. Christoph von Furer-Haimendorf, ed. Pp. 168–182. Warminster, England: Aris and Phillips.
Hoole, Francis W.
1976 Politics and Budgeting in the World Health Organization. Bloomington: Indiana University Press.

Jones, Rex L.
1976 Spirit Possession and Society in Nepal. *In* Spirit Possession in the Nepal Himalayas. John T. Hitchcock and Rex L. Jones, eds. Pp. 1–12. New Delhi: Vikas Publishing House.

Jones, Rex L., and Shirley Kruz Jones
1976 The Himalayan Woman: A Study of Limbu Women in Marriage and Divorce. Palo Alto, Calif.: Mayfield Publishing Company.

Joseph, Stephen C.
1980 Outline of National Primary Care System Development: A Framework for Donor Involvement. Social Science and Medicine 140:177–180.

Joseph, Stephen C., and Sharon Sianion Russell
1980 Is Primary Care the Wave of the Future? Social Science and Medicine 140:137–144.

Joshi, Bhuwanlal, and Leo E. Rose
1966 Democratic Innovations in Nepal: A Case Study of Political Acculturation. Berkeley and Los Angeles: University of California Press.

Joshi, Nanda Lall
1973 Evolution of Public Administration in Nepal. Kathmandu: Center for Economic Development and Administration.

Justice, Judithanne
1981 International Planning and Health: An Anthropological Case Study of Nepal. Ph.D. Dissertation, University of California, Berkeley.
1983 The Invisible Worker: The Role of the Peon in Nepal's Health Service. Social Science and Medicine 17(14): 967–970.
1984 Can Socio-Cultural Information Improve Health Planning? A Case Study of Nepal's Assistant Nurse Midwife. Social Science and Medicine 19(3): 193–198.

Kessavalu, P. G.
1976 Development of Health Services in Nepal. Assignment Report, September 1973–June 1976. WHO Project: NEP SHS 001. SEA/PHA/174. New Delhi: South-East Asia Region, World Health Organization.

King, Maurice, ed.
1966 Medical Care in Developing Countries: A Symposium from Makerere. Nairobi: Oxford University Press.

King, Maurice, Felicity King, and Soebagio Martodipoero
1978 Primary Child Care: A Manual for Health Workers. Oxford: Oxford University Press.

Klee, Linnea
1980 The Anthropologist in the Market-Place. Contract Consulting and the Culture of Washington. San Francisco: University of California. Unpublished manuscript.

Kramer, Roger G.
1979 Country Demographic Profiles: Nepal (ISP-DP-2). Washington, D.C.: U.S. Dept. of Commerce, Bureau of Census.

Lathem, Willoughby, ed.
1979 The Future of Academic Community Medicine in Developing Countries. New York: Praeger Publishers.

Macdonald, Alexander W.
1975 The Healer in the Nepalese World. In Essays on the Ethnology of Nepal and South-Asia. Alexander W. Macdonald, ed. Pp. 113–128. Kathmandu: Ratna Pustak Bhandar.

Macfarlane, Alan
1976 Resources and Population: A Study of the Gurungs of Nepal. Cambridge: Cambridge University Press.

Mahler, Halfdan
1978 Primary Health Care: Justice in Health. World Health (May): 3.

Mamdani, Mahmood
1972 The Myth of Population Control: Family, Caste, and Class in an Indian Village. New York: Monthly Review Press.

Mburu, F. M.
1981 Implications of the Ideology and Implementation of Health Policy in a Developing Country. Social Science and Medicine 15A: 17–24.

Messerschmidt, Donald A.
1976 The Gurungs of Nepal: Conflict and Change in a Village Society. Warminster, England: Aris and Phillips.
1981 Nogar and Other Traditional Forms of Cooperation in Nepal: Significance for Development. Human Organization 40 (1): 40–47.

Michl, Wolf
1974 Shamanism Among the Chantel of the Dhaulagiri Zone. In The Anthropology of Nepal. Christoph von Furer-Haimendorf, ed. Pp. 223–231. Warminster: Aris and Phillips.

Mihaly, Eugene Bramer
1965 Foreign Aid and Politics in Nepal: A Case Study. London: Oxford University Press.

Miller, Casper J.
1979 Faith-Healers in the Himalayas. Kathmandu: Centre for Nepal and Asian Studies.

Miro, Carmen A., and Joseph E. Potter
  1980 Social Science and Development Policy: The Potential Impact of Population Research. Population and Development Review 6(3): 421–437.
Muni, S. D., ed.
  1977 Nepal: An Assertive Monarchy. New Delhi: Chetana Publications.
Nader, Laura
  1974 Up the Anthropologist: Perspectives Gained from Studying Up. In Reinventing Anthropology. Dell Hymes, ed. Pp. 284–311. New York: Vintage Books.
Nath, Tribhuvan
  1975 The Nepalese Dilemma. New Delhi: Sterling Publishers.
Navarro, Vicente
  1974 The Underdevelopment of Health or the Health of Underdevelopment: An Analysis of the Distribution of Human Health Resources in Latin America. International Journal of Health Services 4(1): 5–26.
Nepal-Berkeley Family Planning/Maternal and Child Health Project
  1975 Workshop-Conference on Population, Family Planning, and Development in Nepal. Berkeley: Nepal-University of California, Family Planning/Maternal and Child Health Project and His Majesty's Government of Nepal-Family Planning/Maternal and Child Health Project.
  1976 Conference on the Implementation of Population Policies. Jointly Sponsored by: Population Policies Coordination Board, Nepal; Ministry of Health; University of California, Berkeley-Family Planning/Maternal and Child Health Project in Nepal.
Nepal. Community Health and Integration Division
  1979a Community Volunteer Health Manual. Draft prepared for Workshop, CEDA, Tribhuvan University, March.
  1979b Expanded Programme of Immunization Within the Integrated Community Health Project: Programme and Operations Reference Manual. Kathmandu: Ministry of Health, His Majesty's Government.
Nepal. Department of Health Services
  1976 Project Formulation for Basic Health Services. Kathmandu: Ministry of Health, His Majesty's Government.
  1977 Annual Report of the Integrated Community Health Division 2033–34 (1976–78). Kathmandu: Ministry of Health, His Majesty's Government.
  1978a Annual Report of the Integrated Community Health Di-

vision 2034–35 (1977–78). Kathmandu: Ministry of Health, His Majesty's Government.

1978b Annual Targets of Center and Districts F.Y. 2034/035. Kathmandu: Community Health and Integration Division, Ministry of Health, His Majesty's Government.

1978c Preliminary Evaluation of Ayurvedic Drugs Utilization in Integrated Health Posts. Kathmandu: Ministry of Health, His Majesty's Government.

Nepal. Department of Medicinal Plants
1970 Medicinal Plants of Nepal. Kathmandu: Ministry of Forests, His Majesty's Government.

Nepal. Directorate of Health Services
1969 A Report on Health and Health Administration in Nepal. Kathmandu: Ministry of Health, His Majesty's Government.

Nepal. Institute of Medicine
1979 Health Manpower Directory 2036 (1979). Kathmandu: Research Division, Institute of Medicine, Tribhuvan University.

Nepal. Janchbujh Kendra
1976 Long-Term Health Plan. Kathmandu: Royal Palace, His Majesty's Government.

Nepal. Ministry of Health
1979 Mid-Term Health Review 2035: Research and Evaluation of Health and Health Services Mid-Fifth Plan Period (2031–2036). Kathmandu: Ministry of Health, His Majesty's Government.

Nepal. National Planning Commission
1979 Basic Principles of the Sixth Plan (1980–1985). Kathmandu: His Majesty's Government.

Nepal. Planning Unit, Ministry of Health
1979 Nepal: Country Health Programming Exercise for the Preparation of the Sixth Plan: Programme Proposals for Health Ministry (1980–85). Kathmandu: Ministry of Health, His Majesty's Government.

1980 Planning for Health Manpower. Kathmandu: Ministry/Department of Health and Institute of Medicine, His Majesty's Government.

Nepali, Gopal Singh
1965 The Newars: An Ethno-Sociological Study of a Himalyan Community. Bombay: United Asia Publications.

New Era
1978 Health Survey: Operation Report for Mid-Term Review of the Five Year Health Plan. Kathmandu.

1981 Children of Nepal: A Situational Analysis. Kathmandu: UNICEF.

Newell, Kenneth W.
1975 Health By the People. Geneva: World Health Organization.
Noronha, Raymond
1977 The Anthropologist as Practioner. Anthropological Quarterly 50:211–16.
Okada, Ferdinand E.
1976 Notes on Two Shaman-Curers in Kathmandu. Contributions to Nepalese Studies 3 (Special Issue): 107–112.
Padfield, Nigel W.
1978 Nepal: Kosi Hill Area Rural Development Programme. Report of the Health Advisor. Kathmandu: Ministry of Overseas Development, Britain.
Panday, Devendra Raj
1983 Foreign Aid in Nepal's Development: An Overview. Paper presented at seminar on "Foreign Aid and Development in Nepal," October 4–5, 1983. Kathmandu: Integrated Development Systems.
Parker, Robert L., et al.
1979 Self-Care in Rural Areas of India and Nepal. Culture, Medicine and Psychiatry 3:3–28.
Pitt, David C., ed.
1976 Development from Below: Anthropologists and Development Situations. The Hague: Mouton.
Post, Glenn L., and Ramesh Man Shrestha
1979 Surkhet District Community Health Survey 1978. Kathmandu: Nepal/Canada Surkhet Assistant Health Worker Training Center Project, Institute of Medicine, Tribhuvan University.
Pradhan, Prachanda
1976 Public Administration in Nepal. Kathmandu: Tribhuvan University Press.
Rajbhandari, Bharat Lall
1973 Foreign Assistance in Nepal: A Brief Review. Kathmandu: Mrs. Savitri Devi Rajbhandari.
Ralston, Lenore, James Anderson, and Elizabeth Colson
1983 Voluntary Efforts in Decentralized Management: Opportunities and Constraints in Rural Development. Berkeley: Institute of International Studies, University of California.
Rana, Pashupati Shumshere J. B., and Kamal P. Malla, eds.
1973 Nepal in Perspective. Kathmandu: Centre for Economic Development and Administration.
Ratcliffe, John
1978 Social Justice and the Demographic Transition: Lessons from

India's Kerala State. International Journal of Health Services 8(1): 123–143.

Reed, Horace B., and Mary J. Reed
1968 Nepal in Transition: Educational Innovation. Pittsburgh: University of Pittsburgh Press.

Regmi, Mahesh C.
1962 Recent Land Reform Programs in Nepal. Asian Survey 1(7): 32–38.
1976 Landownership in Nepal. Berkeley, Los Angeles, London: University of California Press.
1977–1981 Nepal Press Digest 21–25. Kathmandu.
1978 Thatched Huts and Stucco Palaces: Peasants and Landlords in Nineteenth-Century Nepal. New Delhi: Vikas Publishing House.

Rein, Martin
1976 Social Science and Social Policy. New York: Penguin.

Rifkin, Susan B.
1977 Politics in Health on a Social Scale. Far Eastern Economic Review (25 November): 33–35.

Rose, Leo E.
1971 Nepal: Strategy for Survival. Berkeley, Los Angeles, London: University of California Press.

Rose, Leo E., and Margaret W. Fisher
1970 The Politics of Nepal: Persistence and Change in an Asian Monarchy. Ithaca: Cornell University Press.

Rose, Leo E., and Martin Landau
1977 Bureaucratic Politics and Development in Nepal. In Leadership in South Asia. B. N. Pandey, ed. Pp. 41–45. New Delhi: Vikas Publishing House.

Rose, Leo E., and John T. Scholz
1980 Nepal: Profile of a Himalayan Kingdom. Boulder, Col.: Westview Press.

Rosen, Charles B.
1980 The Dynamics of Provincial Administration in Haile Selassie's Ethiopia: 1930–1974. In Hierarchy and Society: Anthropological Perspective on Bureaucracy. Gerald M. Britan and Ronald Cohen, eds. Pp. 89–122. Philadelphia: Institute for the Study of Human Issues, Inc.

Sanday, Peggy Reeves, ed.
1976 Anthropology and the Public Interest: Fieldwork and Theory. New York: Academic Press.

Schensul, Stephen, and Jean Schensul
   1978 Advocacy and Applied Anthropology. *In* Social Scientists as
   Advocates. G. Weber and G. McCall, eds. Beverly Hills: Sage.
Schloss, Aran
   1977 Transportation and Development in Nepal: An Inquiry into
   the Dynamic of Development and Administration and Development Policy Making. Ph.D. Dissertation, University of California, Berkeley.
   1980 Making Planning Relevant: Nepal's Experience, 1968–1976.
   Asian Survey 10:1008–1022.
Scholz, John Thomas
   1977 Policy Processes and Rural Development: A Study of Land
   Reform in Nepal. Ph.D. Dissertation, University of California,
   Berkeley.
   1981 Central Commands and Local Political Cultures: The Prob-
   lem of Linkage in Nepal. Unpublished manuscript.
Scholz, John T., and Leo E. Rose
   1980 Trying to Control the Policy Process. Contributions to Asian
   Studies 14:87–102.
Scott, James C.
   1972 Comparative Political Corruption. Englewood Cliffs, N.J.:
   Prentice-Hall.
Shah, Moin, Mathura P. Shrestha, and Marilyn Campbell
   1978 Rural Health Needs: Report of a Seminar Held at Pokhara,
   Nepal, 6–12 October 1977. Ottawa: International Development
   Research Council.
Shah, Moin, Mathura Shrestha, and Robert Parker
   1978 Rural Health Needs. Study No. 1. Report of a Study in the
   Primary Health Care Unit (District) of Tanahu, Nepal. Kath-
   mandu: Institute of Medicine, Tribhuvan University.
   1979 Rural Health Needs. Study No. 2. Report of a Study in the
   Primary Health Care Unit (District) of Dhankuta, Nepal. Kath-
   mandu: Institute of Medicine, Tribhuvan University.
   1980 Rural Health Needs. Study No. 3. Report of a Study in the
   Primary Health Care Unit (District) of Nuwakot, Nepal. Kathmandu: Institute of Medicine, Tribhuvan University.
   1981 Rural Health Needs. Study No. 5. Report of a Study in the
   Primary Health Care Unit (District) of Bara, Nepal. Kathmandu:
   Institute of Medicine, Tribhuvan University.
Shaha, Rishikesh
   1975a An Introduction to Nepal. Kathmandu: Ratna Pustak
   Bhandar.

1975*b* Nepali Politics: Retrospect and Prospect. Delhi: Oxford University Press.

Shakow, Alexander
1980 The Policy Perspective: Anthropology in the Agency for International Development. Paper presented at the 79th Meeting of the American Anthropological Association, Washington, D.C., December.

Sharma, Prayag Raj, ed.
1974 Social Science in Nepal. Kathmandu: Tribhuvan University Press.

Shrestha, Bihari
1983 Technical Assistance and Growth of Administrative Capacity in Nepal. *In* Foreign Aid and Development in Nepal. Proceedings of a Seminar (October 4–5, 1983). Pp. 219–250. Kathmandu: Integrated Development Systems.

Shrestha, Mangal Krishna
1975 Public Administration in Nepal. Kathmandu: Educational Enterprise.

Sikkel, A.
1979 Draft Report of the UNFPA Population Needs Assessment Mission to Nepal. Kathmandu: United Nations Fund for Population Activities.

Sommer, John G.
1977 Beyond Charity: U.S. Voluntary Aid for a Changing Third World. Washington, D.C.: Overseas Development Council.

Stablein, William
1973 A Medical-Cultural System Among the Tibetan and Newar Buddhists: Ceremonial Medicine. Kailash 1(3): 193–202.
1976*a* A Descriptive Analysis of the Content of Nepalese Buddhist Pujas as a Medical Cultural System with References to Tibetan Parallels. *In* The Realm of the Extrahuman: Ideas and Actions. Agehanada Barati, ed. Pp. 165–173. The Hague: Mouton.
1976*b* A Transubstantiated Health Clinic in Nepal: A Model for the Future. *In* Medical Anthropology. F. X. Grollig and H. B. Haley, eds. Pp. 403–411. The Hague: Mouton.
1976*c* Mahakala Neo-shaman: Master of the Ritual. *In* Spirit Possession in the Nepal Himalayas. John T. Hitchcock and Rex L. Jones, eds. Pp. 361–375. New Delhi: Vikas Publishing House.
1976*d* Tantric Medicine and Ritual Blessings. *In* The Tibet Journal: Newark Museum Tibetan Symposium Papers 1(3/4): 55–69.

Stiller, Ludwig
1973 The Rise of the House of Gorkha: A Study of the Unification of Nepal 1768–1816. Kathmandu: Patna Jesuit Society.
1976 The Silent Cry: The People of Nepal 1816–29. Kathmandu: Sahayogi Prakashan.
Stiller, Ludwig, S.J., and Ram Prakash Yadav
1979 Planning for People: A Study of Nepal's Planning Experience. Kathmandu: Sahayogi Prakashan.
Stone, Linda
1976 Concepts of Illness and Curing in a Central Nepal Village. Contributions to Nepalese Studies 3 (Special Issue): 55–80.
Taylor, Carl E.
1978 Development and the Transition to Global Health. Medical Anthropology 2(2): 59–70.
1979 Changing Patterns in International Health: Motivation and Relationships. American Journal of Public Health 69(8): 803–808.
Teas, Jane, Chandra Gurung, and Sumitra Manandhar
1977 Cultural Considerations Important in the Choice Between Ayurvedic and Modern Medical Treatment in Kathmandu. Paper presented at the 76th Meeting of the American Anthropological Association, Houston, 30 December.
Tendler, Judith
1975 Inside Foreign Aid. Baltimore: Johns Hopkins University Press.
Thapa, Bhekh Bahadur
1981 Personal communication, 18 August.
Thapa, Rita
1979 Proposal for National Diarrhoeal Diseases Control Program: Nepal. Kathmandu: Community Health and Integration Division, Ministry of Health, His Majesty's Government of Nepal.
Thapa, Rita, Kalyan Mani Dixit, and Duane L. Smith
1977 Primary Health Care in the Nepalese Context. Kathmandu: Eighth All Nepal Medical Conference.
United Nations Children's Fund
1978 Annual Report on Nepal. Kathmandu: UNICEF.
1980 Status of Children in Nepal: A Research Project. Kathmandu: Child Welfare Co-ordination Committee, UNICEF.
United Nations Development Programme
1978 Primary Health Support Services Programme. Draft Project Document. Kathmandu: United Nations Development Programme.

1979a List of Personnel of the United Nations Organization and Its Specialized Agencies in Nepal. Kathmandu: United Nations Development Programme.

1979b The Resident Representative's Annual Report on Development Assistance to Nepal: Mid 1977–Mid 1978. Kathmandu: United Nations Development Programme.

United Nations Fund for Population Activities

1978 Support to Family Planning and Maternal Child Health Services in Nepal Through the FP/MCH Project and the Integrated Community Health Services. Project number: NEP/74/PO2/II/B. Kathmandu: UNFPA.

1979 Background Paper for Country Needs Assessment Mission. Kathmandu: UNFPA.

United States Agency for International Development

1970 Key Problems Impeding Modernization of Developing Countries: The Health Issues. Washington: USAID.

1972a AID Advisors and Counterparts. Relationships Between Foreign Technical Assistance Experts and Host Country Colleagues. AID Bibliography Series: Technical Assistance Methodology No. 1. Washington: USAID.

1972b Twenty Years of Nepalese-American Cooperation: A Summary of American Aid to Nepal 1951–1971. Washington: USAID.

1976 Project Paper: Integrated Health Services-Nepal. No. 367-11-590-126. Kathmandu: USAID/Nepal.

1977 Workshop on the Role of Anthropology in AID, 27 May. Washington: USAID.

1980a Health Sector Policy Paper. Washington: USAID.

1980b Nepal Project Paper: Integrated Rural Health and Family Planning Services Project (IRH/FP). Project No. 367-0135. Kathmandu: USAID/Nepal.

United States Agency for International Development, World Health Organization, His Majesty's Government of Nepal.

1975 Report on the Evaluation of Basic Health Services in Nepal. Kathmandu: USAID.

Unseem, John

1966 Work Patterns of Americans in India. The Annals of the American Academy of Political and Social Science (November): 146–156.

Veney, James

1979 Nepal Mid-Term Review. Report to the Planning Unit, Health Ministry, HMG Nepal on an Evaluation of the M.T.R. Process. Kathmandu: WHO.

Verderese, Maria de Lourdes
1974 The Traditional Birth Attendant in Maternal and Child Health and Family Planning. A Guide for Her Training and Utilization. Geneva: World Health Organization.
Voulgaropoulos, Emmanuel
1977 Foreign Aid: Asset or Liability? Far Eastern Economic Review (25 November): 35–37.
Wake, C. J.
1976 Health Services and Some Cultural Factors in Eastern Nepal. Contributions to Nepalese Studies 3: 113–126.
Wallace, Anthony, F. C.
1976 Some Reflections on the Contributions of Anthropologists to Public Policy. In Anthropology and the Public Interest. Peggy Sanday, ed. Pp. 3–14. New York: Academic Press.
Wallman, Sandra, ed.
1977 Perceptions of Development. London: Cambridge University Press.
Walt, Gill, and Patrick Vaughan
1981 An Introduction to the Primary Health Care Approach In Developing Countries: A Review with Selected Annotated References. Publication No. 13. London: Ross Institute of Tropical Hygiene.
Watters, David E.
1975 Siberian Shamanistic Traditions Among the Kahm-Magars of Nepal. Contributions to Nepalese Studies 2(1): 124–68.
Werner, David
1977 Where There Is No Doctor: A Village Health Care Handbook. Palo Alto, Calif.: Hesperian Foundation.
Wildavsky, Aaron
1972 Why Planning Fails in Nepal. Administrative Science Quarterly 14(4): 508–528.
Willner, Dorothy
1980 For Whom the Bell Tolls: Anthropologists Advising on Public Policy. American Anthropologist 82(1): 79–94.
World Bank
1975 Health Sector Policy Paper. Washington, D.C.: World Bank.
1978 Nepal Country Economic Memorandum. Report No. 1873a-NEP. Washington, D.C.: World Bank.
1979 Bank Lending for Health. Washington, D.C.: World Bank.
World Health Organization
1958 The First Ten Years of the World Health Organization. Geneva: World Health Organization.

1968 The Second Ten Years of the World Health Organization 1958–1967. Geneva: World Health Organization.

1973 Report on a Workshop on the Role of Social and Cultural Factors in Planning and Programming for Infant Health Care held in Kathmandu from 25 September to 2 October 1973. WHO Project: SEARO 0130. SEA/HE/67. New Delhi: Regional Office for South-Asia, WHO.

1974 Country Health Programming Nepal. Volume I: Programme Proposals 1975–76 to 1979–80. Volume II: Country Profile. Kathmandu: Department of Health, Ministry of Health, His Majesty's Government of Nepal.

1978 A Decade of Health Development in South-East Asia 1968–1977. New Delhi: Regional Office for South-East Asia, WHO.

1979 Country Profile Nepal. Kathmandu: World Health Organization.

1984 Health for All: One Common Cause. Geneva: World Health Organization.

World Health Organization and UNICEF

1978 Primary Health Care: Alma-Ata 1978. Report of the International Conference on Primary Health Care Alma-Ata, USSR, 6–12 September. Geneva: World Health Organization.

Worth, Robert N., and Narayan K. Shaha

1969 Nepal Health Survey 1965–1966. Honolulu: University of Hawaii Press.

Index

Accountability, 32, 64
Acupuncture, 8
Advisors. *See* Foreign advisors
Age, of health post staff, 96
Agriculture, 5, 84, 97
AID. *See* United States Agency for International Development (USAID)
Allopathic medicine, 8, 47, 93–95, 96, 97, 107, 108. *See also* Medical doctors; Medicines
Alma Ata conference, 59–60, 74
Animal care, 97
ANMs. *See* Assistant nurse-midwives
"Annual Report for 2034–35 (1977–78)," 124
"Annual Targets of Center and Districts for Fiscal Year 2034/035 (1977/78)," 123
Anthropologist, 2, 4–5, 14, 113, 134–139, 150, 154, 170, 173
Anthropology, Health, and Development, 137
Assistant health workers, 55, 88, 89–90, 100, 101
Assistant nurse-midwives (ANMs), 55, 88, 90–91, 98, 100, 106, 139–150, 167–169, 173, 174
Ayurvedic doctors, 8, 96, 99

Bangladesh, 7, 64
Bara, 12, 54–56
"Barefoot doctor," 60, 105
Basic health services, 1, 2, 52–59, 70. *See also* Integrated Basic Health Services
Bilateral agencies, 24, 25, 26, 48, 75, 119, 171. *See also individual agencies*
Birganj, 32
Bir Hospital, 102
Birthrate, 7–8
Blood samples, 97
Britain, 34
Britain Nepal Medical Trust (BNMT), 11, 39, 95, 108–109, 153, 171
Buddhists, 7, 8
Budgets: international aid, 25, 27, 38, 47–48, 50, 114; for Nepali bureaucrats, 38; Nepali health, 9. *See also* Finances
Bureaucracies, 4–5, 15–45, 104–106, 109, 111, 147–148, 151–154, 170, 171, 172. *See also* Government structure; International donor agencies
Bureaucrats. *See* Foreign advisors; Nepali bureaucrats

Canada, 34
Canadian International Develop-

ment Agency (CIDA), 11, 30–32, 39, 119, 171
Castes, 21, 84, 88, 136
Catholic mission organization, 24
Cement construction, 34–35
Central Secretariat, 16, 17, 30, 148
Chakari system, 21–22
Chief district officers (CDCs), 16, 99
Childhood diseases, 7, 62, 140. See also Maternal and child health
China, 8, 59–60
Chittre, 88–95, 106–107, 110, 153
Chloraquine, 49
Christian missions, 8, 24, 39, 47
Clerks: at district health offices, 98; at health posts, 88, 91
Colonial era, 46–47
Community health volunteer. See Community participation
Community participation, 23–24, 59, 93, 121–122; with community health volunteers, 73, 74–81, 104–109 passim, 161–163; peons and, 104, 105, 107, 109
Conferences, 59–60, 74, 78–79
Construction, of health posts, 34–35, 79, 84, 88, 93
Consultants, 2, 25, 26–29, 30, 32, 35–38, 72, 115, 116, 117, 122, 140, 148, 153. See also Health Associates
Costs. See Finances
Council of Ministers, 17
Country Health Profile on Nepal, 70–71, 116
Country health programming, 63–68, 71
Cuba, 60
Cultural information. See Information; Sociocultural information
Culture, of bureaucracies, 4–5, 14, 20–24, 35–45, 106. See also Bureaucracies; Sociocultural information

Data, 16; analysis, 65, 66, 73, 125; gathering, 56, 65, 72, 133. See also

Information; Sociocultural information; Statistics
DDT, 2, 49, 50
"Declaration of Alma Ata," 60
Department of Health Services, 17, 82–83, 99; and community participation, 75, 78, 109; Division of Integrated Basic Health Services in, 53, 56–57; and health post construction, 35; Indent and Procurement Section of, 43; and information, 120, 124, 126, 131–132; training by, 32
Dhading, 12
Dhais, 8, 91, 145
Dhamis, 8
Dhankuta, 12, 32
Diarrhea, infant, 7, 62, 97, 126
Dieffenback, Alan E., 40
Director-General of Health Services, 17
Diseases, 95; childhood, 7, 62, 140; communicable, 7, 26, 46–47, 48–50, 100, 107. See also Leprosy; Malaria; Smallpox; Tuberculosis; Vertical programs
District health offices, 17, 23, 55, 98–100, 127
District medical officers, 17, 55, 98, 99–100, 144
Districts, 12, 13, 16
Doctors: Ayurvedic, 8, 96, 99. See also Healers; Medical doctors
Donde No Hay Doctor, 78
Donor agencies. See International donor agency
Dooley Foundation, 11, 39, 119, 171
Drugs, allopathic, 8, 81, 92, 93–95, 96, 97, 99, 107, 108, 110, 124, 153. See also Medicines
Dutch government, 34, 95, 171. See also Netherlands

Education, of Nepali bureaucrats, 21. See also Training
Ethnic groups, 7, 20–21, 84, 88, 110, 136

Evaluation, 29, 55, 73, 76, 108, 124, 126–127, 138, 139, 148
Expanded Program of Immunization (EPI), 33, 57, 124

Family, 21–22, 42–43
Family planning, 3, 27, 33, 50–51, 55, 58, 66, 69, 80, 108, 126, 132
Field training, for ANMs, 144, 149–150
Field visits, 12–14, 100, 117–119, 122, 123, 130
Finances: of foreign advisors, 38, 39–40; of government officials, 38, 40; of health post workers, 80, 91; for international aid, 8–9, 10, 25, 27, 32, 33, 38, 41, 47–48, 50, 58–59, 62, 74, 75, 105, 115, 120, 129, 147, 148, 152; per capita, 57
Firewood, 5
First aid training, 106, 107
Food and Agriculture Organization (FAO), 3
Ford Foundation, 24
Foreign advisors, 21, 26, 27–29, 35–43, 44–45, 65, 70, 71, 73, 74, 76, 77, 104, 130, 135, 136, 148, 152, 153. See also Bureaucracies
Foreign assistance. See Finances; Funding
Forms, for statistics, 124–127
FP/MCH. See Family planning; Maternal and child health
Fuknes, 95
Funding, of international aid, 8–9, 10, 25, 27, 32, 47–48, 50, 75. See also Finances

Geography: of health post organization, 82; Nepal, 5, 6
Government structure, 15–19, 31, 43, 171. See also Ministry of Health; Nepali bureaucrats

Hall, Douglas E., 40
Healers, 8, 95, 96

Health assistants, 55, 83, 101–102, 110, 131, 143; at Chittre, 88, 89; statistics collection by, 125, 126; at Tate, 84–85, 86
Health Associates, 29, 35–37, 56, 108, 115, 138
Health committees, 79–80
Health inspectors, 17, 55, 83, 98, 99, 100, 128, 129; and community health volunteers, 76–77, 79; field visits by, 130–131
Health Manpower Survey, 105, 141
Health Planning Unit, 35, 70, 71–72, 80
Health posts, 9, 12, 17, 23, 54–55, 82–97, 109–110; ANMs at, 55, 88, 90–91, 141–144, 149; construction of, 34–35, 79, 84, 88, 93; district health offices and, 17, 23, 55, 98–99, 127; field visits to, 117–119, 122, 123, 130; fully integrated, 82, 88–95; health committees and, 12, 79–80, 93; nonintegrated, 82; partially integrated, 82, 83–87; peons at, 83, 85–86, 88, 91, 101–106, 107, 109, 110, 139; statistics collected at, 125–127
Herbal medicine, 8, 95, 96
Hierarchical system, 21–22, 143
Hill Development Project, 34
Hindus, 7, 8, 142
Home Ministry, 16
Homeopathy, 8
Hospitals, 9, 33–34, 48, 95; ANMs in, 141, 149; peons in, 102
Hygiene, 9, 126

ICHP. See Integrated Community Health Program
Immunization, 33, 97
Income per capita, 5–7
Indent and Procurement Section, 43
India, 2–3, 4, 8, 21, 171
Infant diarrheal disease, 7, 62, 97, 126
Infant mortality, 7, 50, 140
Informal networks, 20, 21–22, 23–24, 42–45, 89, 90, 120–122

Information, 2–4, 12, 20, 22, 64, 109, 111–154, 170, 172; analysis of, 66–67, 73; flow of, 111–112, 121, 122–132, 139, 151–152; qualitative, 65; quantitative, 65, 66, 113, 123, 132–133; sources of, 111, 112–122. *See also* Data; Reports; Sociocultural information; Statistics
Institute of Medicine (IOM), 32, 34, 84, 89, 131–132, 146
Integrated Basic Health Services (IBHS), 52–59, 61, 66–67, 69–70
Integrated Community Health Program (ICHP), 3–4, 12, 15, 17, 24–41 passim, 59, 110, 133, 139, 172; community participation and, 59, 74, 75, 76, 77, 78, 79; and district health office/health inspectors, 17, 76–77, 98, 99–100, 127, 129, 130; and health post populations, 82; and information, 115–116, 120, 124, 126, 127, 132; targets for, 123, 127, 132; transfers in, 96, 100; USAID and, 11, 24–38 passim, 74, 75, 108, 109; and VHWs, 83, 108, 109, 110
Integration, 52–53, 62–63, 67, 70, 82, 132, 152; and ANMs, 141. *See also* Integrated Basic Health Services; Integrated Community Health Program
International Conference on PHC, Alma Ata, Soviet Union, 59–60, 74
International donor agencies, 1, 2, 8–12, 15, 17, 21, 24–29, 32, 34, 39, 46–48, 51, 56, 61, 62, 74, 77, 105, 112, 117, 120, 122, 128, 129, 130, 133, 137, 147, 148, 151–154, 171. *See also* Foreign advisors; *individual agencies*
International health agencies. *See* International donor agencies
International Research Development Centre (IDRC), 11
International Women's Year, 147
Isolation era, 21

Janch Bhuj Kendra (Centre for Enquiry and Investigation), 16, 70, 122
Japan, 34, 171
Jhankris, 8, 95
Jharfuknes, 8
Jharnes, 95
Jiri, 34
Johns Hopkins School of Public Health, 71

Kaski, 12, 54, 56
Kathmandu Valley, 12, 101–102
Kings, 76, 94; dynasties of, 20, 21, 22; and government structure, 15, 17, 43

Lalitpur, 12, 97
Landholdings, 7
Languages, 7, 20, 72, 84, 110, 119, 153
League of Nations Health Office, 46
Leprosy, 3, 7, 26, 48, 50, 52, 55, 56, 66, 69–70, 80, 89, 100, 107, 171
Life expectancy, 7
Literacy, 7, 142
Long-Term Health Plan, 16, 70, 73

Mahendra, King, 17
Mahler, Halfdan, 74
Malaria, 1, 3, 7, 9–10, 17, 23, 26, 27, 48, 49–50, 52, 56, 62, 66, 69, 80, 90, 98, 129, 130; Integrated Basic Health Services and, 53, 54, 57, 58; Tate Post and, 84; USAID and, 10, 27, 49, 53; VHWs checking, 91, 107; WHO and, 10, 25, 49
Maternal and child health, 3–4, 7, 50, 55, 58, 62; ANMs and, 55, 140, 145, 149; UNICEF and, 33, 140; VHW checking, 107–108. *See also* Midwives
Maternal mortality, 7, 140
Medical doctors, 8, 9, 17, 34; district, 55, 98, 99–100, planning by, 122; in WHO, 26

Medicine, traditional, 8, 95–96, 170, 172, 173. *See also* Allopathic medicine; Midwives
Medicines: allopathic, 8, 85, 87, 89, 92, 93–95, 96, 102, 107, 108; herbal, 8, 95, 96. *See also* Drugs
Meetings, for information, 119–122, 128–129. *See also* Conferences
Men: among foreign advisors, 39; in health service, 147
Midterm review, 72–73, 105, 128, 144
Midwives, 8, 55, 91, 145–146, 150. *See also* Assistant nurse-midwives
Minister of Health, 17, 78
Ministry of Education, 132
Ministry of Finance, 11, 120
Ministry of Health, 9, 11, 26, 27, 30, 36, 118; and ANMs, 146; and community health volunteers, 75, 77, 78; and Health Planning Unit, 70, 71, 72; and information, 98, 114, 120, 123–124, 127, 132; and integration, 58, 59, 69, 70; and panchayats, 93; and peons, 104–105; structure of, 17–19
Morbidity rates, 7, 126–127. *See also* Diseases
Mortality rates, 7, 50, 126–127, 140
Mosquitoes, malaria-transmitting, 49, 50
Mukhiya (clerk), 88, 91
Multilateral agencies, 5, 24, 48, 112, 171. *See also individual agencies*
Multinational organizations. *See* Multilateral agencies
Muslims, 7

National Panchayat (*Rastriya Panchayat*), 16n, 17, 78
National Fertility Survey, 8
National Planning Commission. *See* Planning Commission
Natural resources, 5
Nepali bureaucrats, 41, 42–45, 113, 115–116, 119–120, 148; education

of, 21; elite, 21–24, 78–79; information flow among, 122–132, 133, 135, 152; and peons, 104; and USAID, 30, 35–36, 37, 38, 113, 114; and WHO, 35, 36, 37, 38. *See also* Bureaucracies
Netherlands, 34, 95, 171. *See also* Dutch government
North Vietnam, 59
Nurses, 9, 144–145. *See also* Assistant nurse-midwives; Public health nurses
Nutrition, 7, 9, 66, 80, 97, 99, 107

Objectives, of foreign aid, 47
Office Internationale d'Hygiene Publique, 46
Oral rehydration fluid, 80, 97, 107, 126, 163
Oxfam, 24

Palace Secretariat, 15–16, 30, 43, 70
Palpa, 12
Pan American Sanitary Bureau, 46
Panchayats, 12, 16–17, 22, 23, 83, 92–93
Parsa, 12
Pathlaiya Training Center, 86
Pensions, for foreign advisors, 39–40
Peons, 83, 101–106, 107, 109, 110, 139, 146–147, 172; at Chittre, 88, 91; at district health offices, at Tate, 83, 85–86
Per diem expense allowances, 40, 76, 130
Physicians. *See* Medical doctors
Planners, health, 1, 2, 3, 4, 10, 14, 73, 111, 135–139, 146–147, 151, 153–154
Planning Commission, 11, 72, 75, 121, 123, 124, 127; and community participation, 75, 77, 78, 80; and Health Planning Unit, 71, 72
Planning process, 2, 14, 63–81, 123,

134, 152; information for, 111–154 (*see also* Information)
Pokhara, 32, 118
Policy, health, 3, 11, 14, 17, 29–30, 48, 59, 105, 111, 147, 151–152
Policy implementation, 16, 30, 43
Policy making, 15–16, 30, 43, 61–63, 147
Political elites, 21–24, 78–79
Political parties, 23
Population: of foreign advisors, 38–39; in health post service area, 82, 84; Nepal, 5, 22, 51; worldwide, 50–51
Preventive medicine, 47, 97
Primary health care (PHC), 2, 4, 17, 59–63, 74, 96, 129, 140, 146, 152
Private organizations, 24, 39, 48, 120; religious, 8, 12, 24, 39, 47, 48; voluntary group, 24, 48, 75, 95, 108–109, 153, 171
Project chief, 17, 120
Project formulations, 69–70, 73, 115–116
Protestant mission organizations, 24, 47
Public health nurses (PHNs), 100, 144–145

Quarantine movement, 46

Ranas, 21, 22
Rapti Valley, 49
Rautahat, 12
Red Cross, Nepal, 75
Regionalism, 20
Registers, 124–125
Rehydration therapy. *See* Oral rehydration fluid
Religion, in Nepal, 7
Religious missions, 8, 12, 24, 39, 47, 48, 171
Reports: anthropologists', 135, 138; donor agency, 55–56, 70–71, 112–116; district/health post, 98, 99, 126–127, 130–131; government, 55–56, 122

Residence, of foreign advisors, 39
Responsibility, among Nepali bureaucrats, 43
Rising Nepal, 121–122
Rockefeller Foundation, 24
Rural areas, 9, 10, 52–53, 60–61, 67, 79, 82–110; ANMs in, 55, 88, 90–91, 141, 142–144, 146, 149–150; information on, 30, 67, 72–73, 109, 117–119, 121, 122–123, 130, 131, 135, 146–147, 151–153; public health nurses in, 145. *See also* Health posts

Salaries: of foreign advisors, 39, 40; of *mukhiyas*, 91; of village health workers, 80
Sanitation, 9, 66, 80
Sankhuwasabha, 12, 108–109
Save the Children, 24, 39, 119, 171
Scientific management, 64
Secretary of Health, 17, 37, 121
Shah, Prithvi Narayan, 20
Shah dynasty, 20, 21
Shortages, of health post supplies, 85, 93–95, 110
Siklis, 122
Smallpox, 1, 3, 23, 25, 33, 48, 50, 57, 66, 69; VHW checking, 107; WHO and, 25, 57
Social life, of foreign advisors, 41, 121
Social scientists, 2, 3, 11, 116, 137, 139
Social Service Coordination Committee, 77
Social soundness analysis, 116, 137, 154
Social status, 21–22, 96, 103, 143–144. *See also* Castes; Ethnic groups
Sociocultural information (Nepal), 5–8, 20–24, 42–45, 111, 116, 133, 134–154; *See also* Information; Rural areas
"Source and force," 43–44, 89, 90
Soviet Union, 8
Statistics, 7n, 133, 138, 151; gather-

ing of, 65–66, 72–73, 99, 124–128; reports of, 98, 99, 126–127, 130–131
Stiller, Ludwig S. J., 40
Success, 44
Sudenis, 8, 91, 145
Supervision, 29, 36, 54–55, 80, 83, 85, 86, 98, 110, 126, 129–131, 144
Supplies, 85, 93–95, 107, 129, 131. See also Drugs; Medicines
Surkhet, 12, 32
Swiss Association for Technical Assistance (SATA), 34, 119, 171
Switzerland, 34

Target system, 65, 66, 122–124, 125, 127, 131, 132
Tate, 83–87, 94, 110
Terai, 12; ANMs in, 143; community participation in, 76; field visits to, 130; health post populations in, 82; Integrated Basic Health Services in, 54, 56, 57; malaria in, 49, 57
Thailand, 64
Tibetan medicine, 8
Traditional birth attendants (TBAs), 145–146, 150, 172. See also Midwives
Training, 32, 34, 48, 100, 105, 131; for ANMs, 140–141, 144, 146, 149; for community health volunteers, 75–77, 78, 106–107; for health assistants, 84, 89, 110; for village health workers, 86
Tribhuvan University, 78
Tuberculosis, 3, 7, 17, 48, 50, 56, 66, 69, 80, 86, 95, 107

UNFPA. See United Nations Fund for Population Activities
UNICEF. See United Nations Children's Fund
United Mission to Nepal, 97, 171
United Nations, 2, 21, 24, 39, 40, 75, 140, 171
United Nations Children's Fund (UNICEF), 3, 11, 72, 99, 118, 119, 129, 134, 137, 171; and ANMs, 140, 147; and community participation, 74, 76; and integrated basic health services, 52, 53, 57; and primary health care, 59, 74; supplies provided by, 94; and vertical programs, 33, 57
United Nations Development Program (UNDP), 11, 38, 171
United Nations Fund for Population Activities (UNFPA), 32, 72, 75–76, 113, 115, 116, 171
United States, 8, 21, 34, 71
United States Agency for International Development (USAID), 10, 11, 24, 26–40 passim, 48, 109, 129, 134, 153, 171, 173; and ANMs, 140; anthropologists used by, 137; and community health volunteers, 74, 75; and country health programming, 68; and drug supplies, 95; family planning project of, 27, 33, 50, 172; and Health Planning Unit, 35, 71, 72; and integrated basic health services, 53, 55, 56, 57; and malaria eradication, 10, 27, 49, 53; and midterm review, 73; and reports, 55–56, 113, 114, 116; and VHWs, 108, 109
United States Congress, 26, 52, 113, 116
United States Department of State, 26
USAID. See United States Agency for International Development

Vasectomy, 97, 99
Veks, 54, 82–83
Vertical programs, 3–4, 33, 48–51, 82; and integration, 33, 52, 56–57, 58, 62, 67, 69–70, 124; project formulation with, 69–70. See also Family planning; Malaria; Smallpox
Veterinary services, 97
Village health workers (VHWs), 54–

55, 82, 83, 93–94, 103, 107–109, 110, 139; at Chittre, 88, 91; and community health volunteers, 80–81, 107, 108; job description for, 163–167; statistics collection by, 125–127; at Tate, 83, 85, 86–87
Villages. *See* Rural areas
Voluntary groups, 12, 24, 39, 48, 75, 95, 108–109, 153, 171
Volunteers, community health, 73, 74–81, 104–109 passim, 161–163

Water, polluted, 5, 9
Werner, David, 78
West Germany, 34, 171
Where There Is No Doctor, 78
WHO. *See* World Health Organization
Women, among foreign advisors, 39
Women's roles, ANMs and, 140, 142, 143, 147, 149, 150
World Bank, 11, 34, 137, 171
World Health Organization (WHO),
8, 10, 11, 24, 25–40 passim, 48, 118, 119, 134, 137, 171; and ANMs, 140, 145, 146, 147; anthropologists used by, 137; and community participation, 59, 74, 76, 78, 79; *Country Health Profile* by, 70–71, 116; country health programming by, 63–66, 67, 68; and Health Planning Unit, 35, 71, 72; and integrated basic health services, 52, 53, 55; in malaria eradication campaign, 10, 25, 49; and midterm review, 73; and peons, 104; and project formulation, 69–70; and quarantine movement, 46; and reports, 55, 70–71, 116; and smallpox programs, 25, 57

Yadav, Ram Prakash, 40
Yunani, 8

Zonal commissioner, 16
Zones, 16

COMPARATIVE STUDIES OF HEALTH SYSTEMS
AND MEDICAL CARE

John M. Janzen, *The Quest for Therapy in Lower Zaire*

Paul U. Unschuld, *Medical Ethics in Imperial China: A Study in Historical Anthropology*

Margaret M. Lock, *East Asian Medicine in Urban Japan: Varieties of Medical Experience*

Jeanie Schmit Kayser-Jones, *Old, Alone, and Neglected: Care of the Aged in Scotland and in the United States*

Arthur Kleinman, *Patients and Healers in the Context of Culture: An Exploration of the Borderland between Anthropology, Medicine, and Psychiatry*

Stephen J. Kunitz, *Disease Change and the Role of Medicine: The Navajo Experience*

Carol Laderman, *Wives and Midwives: Childbirth and Nutrition in Rural Malaysia*

Victor G. Rodwin, *The Health Planning Predicament: France, Québec, England, and the United States*

Michael W. Dols and Adil S. Gamal, *Medieval Islamic Medicine: Ibn Ridwān's Treatise "On the Prevention of Bodily Ills in Egypt"*

Leith Mullings, *Therapy, Ideology, and Social Change: Mental Healing in Urban Ghana*

Jean de Kervasdoué, John R. Kimberly, and Victor G. Rodwin, *The End of an Illusion: The Future of Health Policy in Western Industrialized Nations*

Arthur J. Rubel, Carl W. O'Nell, and Rolando Collado-Ardón, *Susto, a Folk Illness*

Paul U. Unschuld, *Medicine in China: A History of Ideas*

Paul U. Unschuld, *Medicine in China: A History of Pharmaceutics*

Glenn Gritzer and Arnold Arluke, *The Making of Rehabilitation: A Political Economy of Medical Specialization, 1890-1980*

Arthur Kleinman and Byron Good, editors, *Culture and Depression: Studies in the Anthropology and Cross-Cultural Psychiatry of Affect and Disorder*

Judith Justice, *Policies, Plans, and People: Culture and Health Development in Nepal*

Paul U. Unschuld, *Nan-ching—The Classic of Difficult Issues*

Viggo Brun and Trond Schumacher, *Traditional Herbal Medicine in Northern Thailand*

Francis Zimmermann, *The Jungle and the Aroma of Meats: An Ecological Theme in Hindu Medicine*

Roger Jeffery, *The Politics of Health in India*

Printed in the United States
203090BV00002B/25-36/A